The Magic of Gooseberries

For Health and Beauty

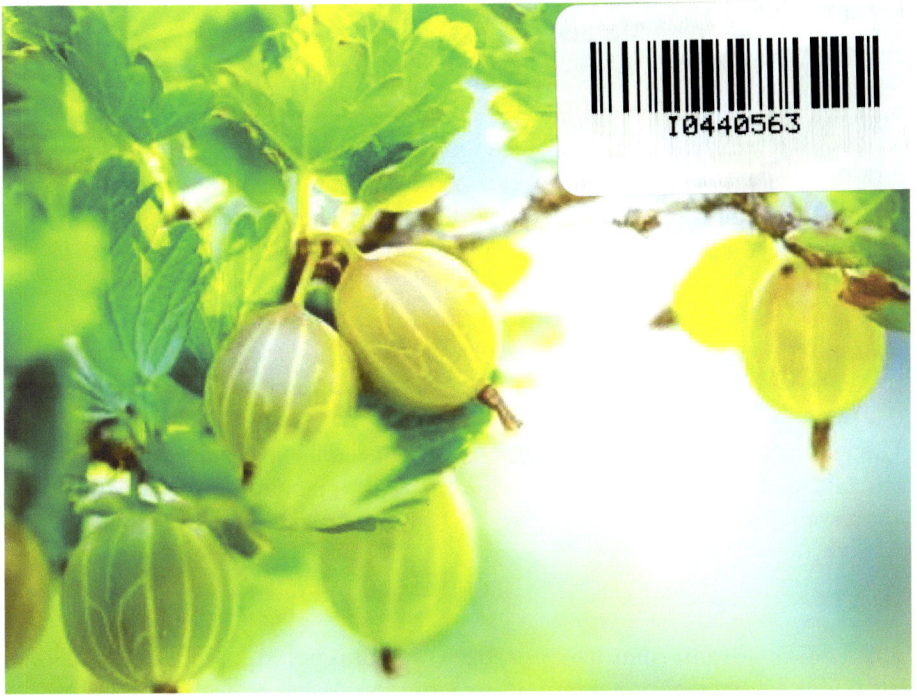

By Dueep Jyot Singh

Natural Remedy Series
Mendon Cottage Books

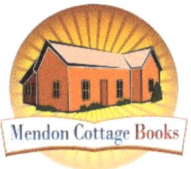

JD-Biz Publishing

Disclaimer

The information is this book is provided for informational purposes only. It is not intended to be used and medical advice or a substitute for proper medical treatment by a qualified health care provider. The information is believed to be accurate as presented based on research by the author.

The contents have not been evaluated by the U.S. Food and Drug Administration or any other Government or Health Organization and the contents in this book are not to be used to treat cure or prevent disease.

The author or publisher is not responsible for the use or safety of any diet, procedure or treatment mentioned in this book. The author or publisher is not responsible for errors or omissions that may exist.

Warning

The Book is for informational purposes only and before taking on any diet, treatment or medical procedure, it is recommended to consult with your primary health care provider.

Our books are available at

1. Amazon.com

2. Barnes and Noble

3. Itunes

4. Kobo

5. Smashwords

6. Google Play Books

Table of Contents

Introduction

Playing gooseberry may be an aphorism to describe an unwanted person, who is not needed in a self-contained and self absorbed group of two, but in reality, the common gooseberry is one of the most precious, wanted and valuable of natural plants.

Gooseberry shrubs can be found all over the world, where the climate has plenty of sun, and the humidity content in the air is high. Native American gooseberries are larger than their Asian counterparts.

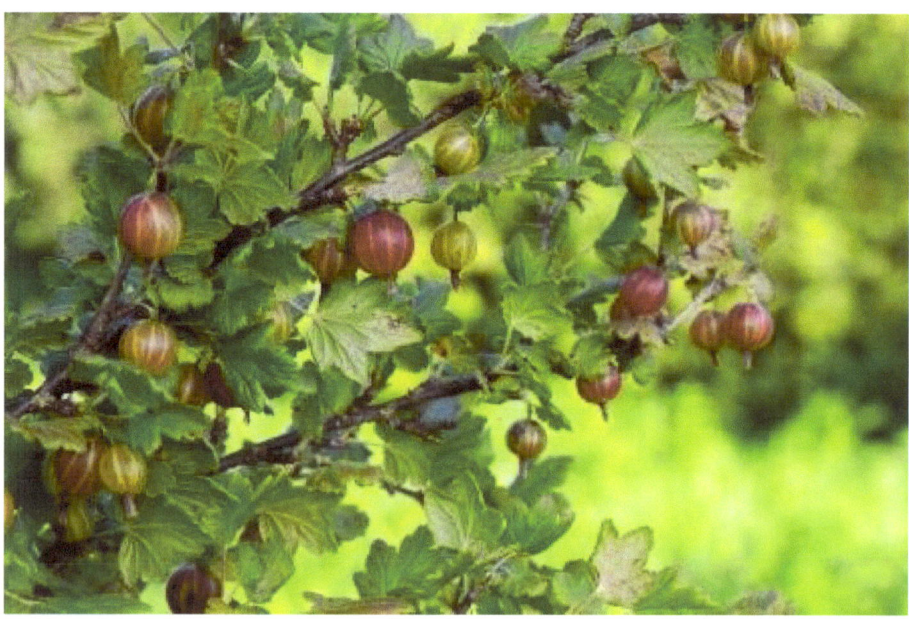

Not only is this an excellent medicinal plant, but it is also well-known for its beautifying qualities. In fact, the ancient sages in the East. Make sure that they had plenty of gooseberries, in their daily diet, because they considered this fruit to be the reason for their longevity, everlasting good health, and youthful looks.

The ancients called this the gift of the gods, and thought that the gods had given the gooseberry to man because even though they could not give him immortality, they could give him longevity in the shape of gooseberries. That is because Indian myth says that this plant grew from a few drops of nectar, dropping on the earth by the gods taking the treasures of the sea, to the heavens. These treasures were obtained by churning the seas by the gods and the demons. Out of them, the nectar of immortality was one.

Gooseberries, also known as Emblica officianalis have long been a religious, and political symbol in India and China.This is the reason why, in ancient Indian history, myth and religious tradition, giving a gooseberry to somebody who you honored and revered was considered to be the prerogative of Kings. The Hindus worship the gooseberry tree, because they consider Lord Vishnu to live in this plant.

Living in South India as a child, I consider myself to have been brought upon gooseberries, because that was what we used to gnaw at school, and best friends used to share their "nellikas" among themselves. Hiding your own supply of gooseberries was considered the height of selfishness and treachery among friends. These gooseberries were of course "purloined" from the gooseberry trees, growing in particularly targeted gardens. It is a wonder how we managed to digest those raw gooseberries, along with raw guavas. And all of us had the lyrics of a very popular song of the time down pat, of which the chorus was – *Nellikai amma illi baa [lit – gooseberry lady, come here…]* We enjoyed the extremely sour taste of gooseberries, when we did not have tamarinds around. And that is why, whenever we had some time to spare, we would be hitting the branches of the deciduous gooseberry tree with a long stick in order to make the gooseberries fall. We could not climb up the tree, because of the vicious thorns surrounding the gooseberries.

The Sanskrit name for gooseberry is amalika from amal- acid. We knew it as Amla, a common name, which is getting to be well known in the West by gooseberry marketers. So if you see that term anywhere in the text, while you are reading, do not worry, it is just our friend, the ubiquitous gooseberry.

So with our pockets full of acidic six striped fruit, we were set for the day. I think this is the reason why all our immunity systems were so strong, as well as our teeth. I have never been to a dentist for teeth problems. QED. That is because of the regular vitamins C intake, day in day out in the shape of gooseberries.

Gooseberries are available all over the world. If you have a gooseberry plant growing in your garden, well, you can consider yourself to be equal to Emperor Asoka The Great, [304 – 232 BCE] who was raised to the status of the Emperor of half a myrobalan from being the Emperor of Jambudwipa(India), when he presented a delegation of Buddhist priests with half a gooseberry as a precious gift.

The fruits of the gooseberry ripen in autumn, if they are allowed to ripen on the branches, by adventurous urchins of the neighborhood. The taste is that astringent, and that is why it is such a popular item for making pickles.

In the South of India, this fruit is normally put in salt water, so that the bitter, sour, as well as astringent taste is reduced considerably. But then, half of the fun of eating a gooseberry goes with the wind, if it has the bland taste.

Since ancient times, sages knew that it had antimicrobial qualities. That is why it was given as a medicine to prevent fevers and diseases, because of its antiviral powers. In fact, people suffering from pancreatitis in ancient times were given plenty of gooseberry, so that the pancreas cells could regenerate.

This is because it is believed that this fruit has cell regeneration properties. Its anti-inflammatory properties, as well as usage as a diabetes preventative or curative, – because it reduces the blood glucose level, – to cure renal diseases have been put into use for millenniums in the East, and are now the basis of scientific research in the West.

In fact, if you are suffering from high cholesterol, and you are living in the East, and you believe in natural remedies, your friendly neighborhood herbalist is going to give you a medicine which is going to consist primarily of Indian gooseberries. You will need to eat one spoon full of it, every morning at breakfast time with a glass full of milk.

Gooseberries have also been known in ancient Greek medicine where the roots, seeds, fruit, bark and dried flowers of this plant are used in different medical preparations.

I am going to give you a recipe later on, for one of the most powerful ancient herbal remedies known to man, for good health and youth. This was written in 500 CE, by a sage named Charaka. According to myth, the son of the serpent King visited the earth, and was horrified to see the ailments troubling human beings. So he decided to be born as the son of a sage, and as he had come to the earth as a spy- Chara ,- he was known as Charaka. He made a compendium of natural remedies, in which he described the way to make Chyavanaprash – a herbal remedy made up of 43 ingredients. Of course, I am going to give you the modern recipe, because some of these rejuvenative items and compounds may not be easily found on the street where you live.

The ancient Chinese called the fruit yuganzi and used it to get rid of any sort of inflammations in the body.

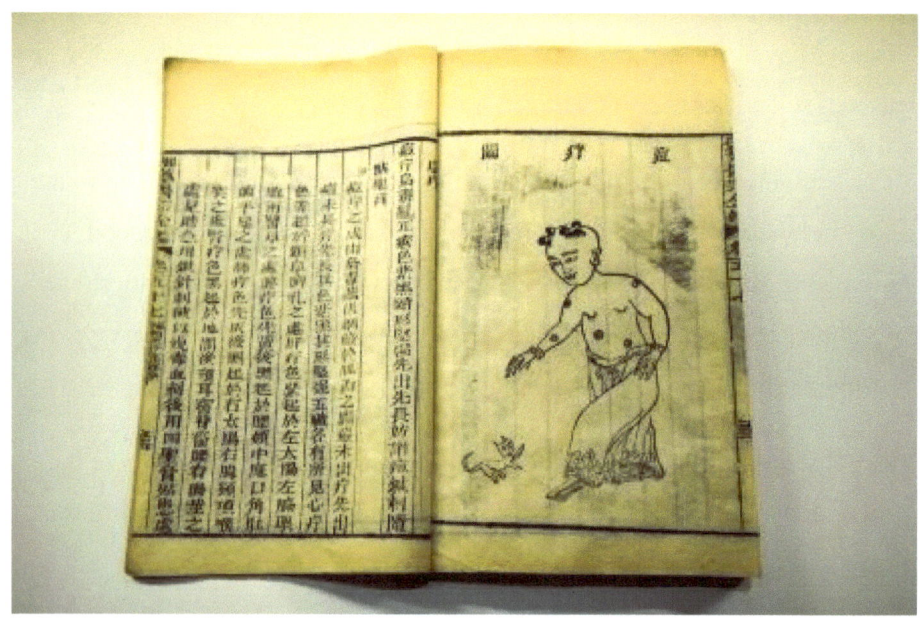

Ancient Chinese medicine books have documented the use of gooseberries.

So now that you know a little bit about the gooseberry, the next chapter is going to tell you all about how to plant it.

How to Grow Gooseberries

I have noticed that gooseberries are very popular in the UK and in other European countries, even though their fan following is growing slowly in the US. Well then, I can only attribute the popularity of this fruit in the UK to those enterprising colonials, who came to India, saw that the natives could not do without gooseberries, wondered why they were so healthy in supposedly insalubrious climes as well as plenty of heat and dust, and then applying the rule of cause and effect, decided that the common gooseberry was the culprit.

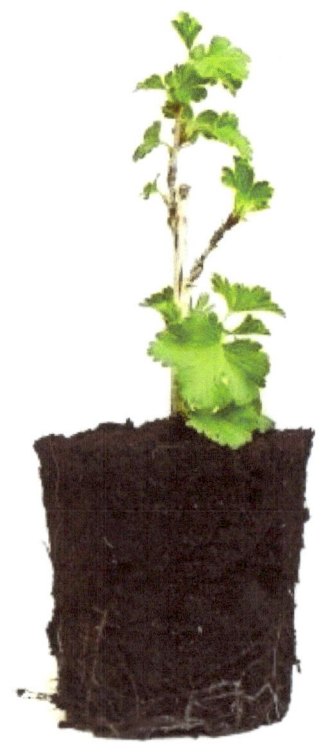

And that is why the gardeners took these gooseberry bushes from the land of endless sunshine to their land of cold winds and gales. Nowadays, you find so many hybrid gooseberry varieties, as well as cultivars, that you are spoilt for choice. A gooseberry needs a humid climate in order to flourish.

Early settlers in the USA brought gooseberry plants from Europe, and hybridized them with the plants they found growing in the generously in their area. The first hybrid was displayed in 1847, at Massachusetts and it was called Houghton. In England, gooseberry wines were almost as popular as dandelion wines, elderberry wines, Apple wines and grape wines.

Gooseberry Varieties

Some of the gooseberry varieties which you may want to look at are 'Achilles', Black Satin' and 'Mt. Ennis', out of the more than 60 varieties and hybrids found all over the world. If you want a little bit of sweetish taste, you can buy the Hybrid Red Jacket.

Fruit production is going to start when the plant is about one year old, depending on the variety. If you live in a hot and sunny climate, these plans are best planted in the shade. They need plenty of rain and moisture so they are definitely not desert plants. However, they do not like waterlogging, so make sure your garden is properly drained, when you water your gooseberries

Heavy clayey moisture retaining soils are better for your gooseberries. You will get juicier fruit.

Gooseberry plants are best planted 6 feet apart, because they need space to grow and flourish. You can either plant them in late fall, if you have a mild winter, or very early in the spring, so that the plan can begin its spring growth as soon as possible.

Shoots that are more than three years old need to be pruned away regularly, so that you can promote the growth of more shoots. These shoots are going to come up annually. So cut the older ones. How do you recognize the older shoots? Older stem bark starts to peel away, as the plant grows. Cut these shoots as close to the ground as possible.

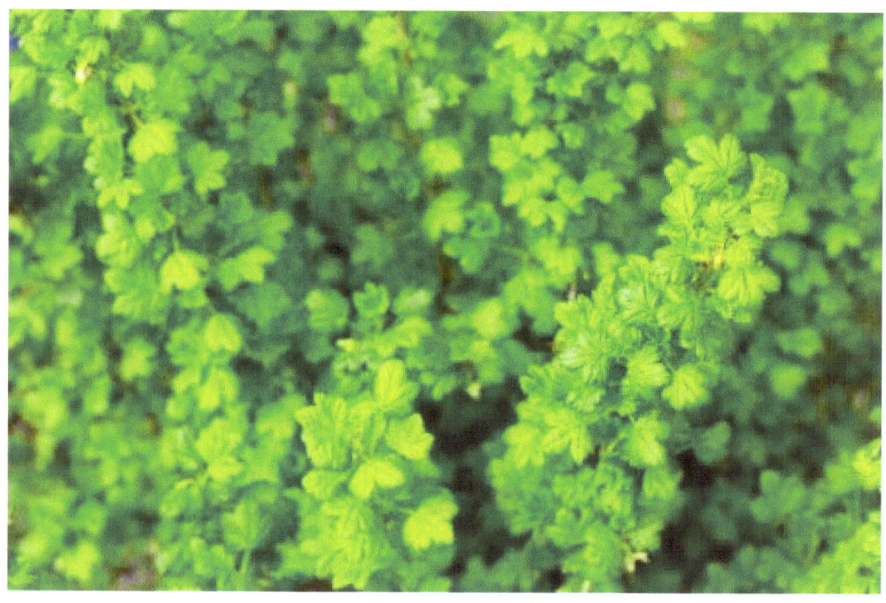

Gooseberry bush with fresh spring leaves

Planting a Single Shoot Gooseberry Tree

I would suggest that you plant a gooseberry tree, so that you do not have to worry about gooseberry branches trailing on the ground. These standard trees are attractive ornamental additions to your garden. How do you train a standard tree? Only one stem needs to be developed on a plant. Tie that stem to a stake. The moment it reaches 3 feet, nip the stem. This is going to promote more plant stem growth and also, you are going to find side branches growing on the stem.

Gooseberry Diseases

Funnily enough, the gooseberries I knew that grew wild in the jungles did not suffer from mildew, leaf rot and other diseases. However, all the gooseberries that I see growing in gardens are rather vulnerable to white patches and leaf spots. That may be possible due to infected plants being brought in from nurseries. So look for disease resistant varieties. You may want to look at antifungals, which can be sprayed on. I normally use a neem oil solution on my plants with half a cup of neem oil to 1 gallon of water.

Gooseberry Cuttings

You can also propagate gooseberry from gooseberry cuttings. Take a cutting about 1 foot long with some leaves on it. Then plant it in a well fertilized shady area. Try planting in the late autumn. I also tried planting stem tips, by burying the tips where they touched the soil, and allowing a new plant to grow from there. This is normally done in the spring.

Gooseberry Harvesting

Harvesting gooseberries is rather tiresome, especially when you do not have thick leather garden gloves. Nevertheless, cover your left hand with a garden glove and use it for holding the branches back. Then use your uncovered right hand to harvest the gooseberries. Many times these gooseberries are best harvested when they are still unripe and allowed to ripen in cold storage.

Gooseberries for Health

The gooseberry, which is a wonder food is an excellent immunity booster do to the presence of many antioxidants that prevent cell damage and promote cell growth. Did you know that it has been assumed that one gooseberry is equal to the amount of vitamins C, which you can get in two oranges, four bananas, eight tomatoes and two Citrons.

Also, the vitamins in gooseberries do not get destroyed, even when you heat them, even though that occurs in other fruits and vegetables. The moment you cook fruit/vegetables in stewing, half of their important minerals, proteins, and other nutrients are lost in the heating process.

Magic Chyavanprash

The original Chyavanprash was made millenniums ago to help keep people healthy. It is either bought in the market, or you can make it right at home. My maternal grandmother ate a spoon full of Chyavanprash at breakfast with a glass of milk, and if she hadn't accidentally slipped in the bathroom and had a hemorage 10 years ago , she would still be going strong at 95+ today.

I am giving you the home recipe for making this rejuvenating compound which is given to children, and old people alike in order to boost their immunity system, keep them healthy, and give them a good start on all round good health.

Children who are suffering from the burden, tests, stress and tension of studies are normally fed Chyavanprash with one teaspoonful of rose jam also known as Gulkand.

Chyavanprash Recipe

Here is the secret recipe for rejuvenation . Ancient sages lived for hundreds of years because they knew the quality of the herbs they ate. These Gooseberry recipes make your skin glow, make you look young, and strengthen your resistance power. Healthy Eldsters in India live well into their 90s because of this recipe. My maternal grandmother ate a spoon full of Chyavanprash at breakfast with a glass of milk, and if she hadn't accidentally slipped in the bathroom and hemorrhaged, a decade ago she would still be going strong at 95 + today.

Put 250 grams of dried Gooseberry powder in 250 g of Gooseberry juice. Add 10 g of slaked lime water . Add two glasses of sugar syrup. Heat this mixture slowly for three hours. Now add 20 g of honey to this thick mixture. This extremely powerful mixture is taken at breakfast time, one spoonful with hot milk.

Gulqand – Rose Jam – Recipe

This is a traditional Persian recipe, which was brought to India by the Moguls. You can call it Rose Jam. It is normally used to combat ailments brought about by summer, especially lethargy, sunstroke, exposure to sun, and other conditions related to heat. Also, if you are stressed out, just have one teaspoonful of this rose jam with milk. It is used in the East as a flavoring agent on desserts, along with Rose sherbet.

So if you are living in Calcutta or California, Sonora or Sydney, Gulkand is the best way in which you can get rid of summer heat.

In ancient Ayurveda and in ancient Persian medicine, doctors used to prescribe Gulkand to all those patients suffering from an imbalance in the pulse. Is your summer sweat foul-smelling, especially in the armpit region?

You may also find yourself sweating excessively if you are stressed and strained.

You need a teaspoonful of Gulkand every day with milk at breakfast, lunch and dinner. In the same way, if you are suffering from hemorrhage or nose bleeding, Gulkand will be suggested to you by an eastern medicine man. The taste is bittersweet and pungent. It is supposed to speed up your metabolism and your digestive system.

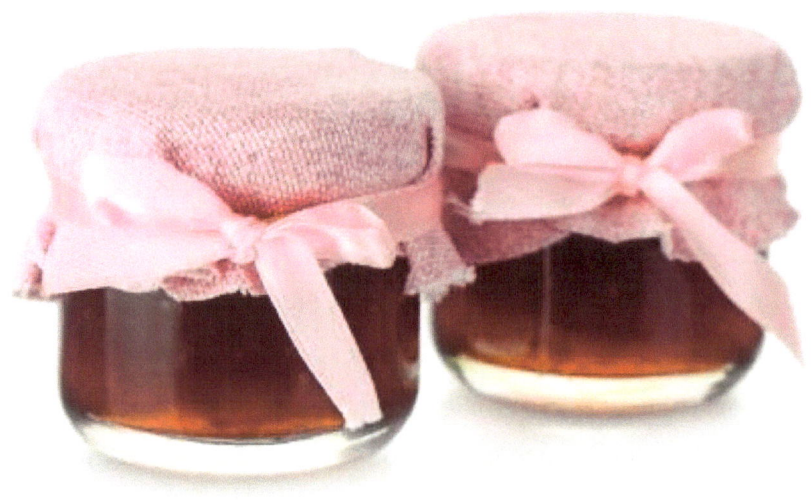

In ancient Greek medicine, it was supposed to be a blood purifier making your skin pimple free and without blemishes.

Also, if you are suffering from stress and strain, this is an excellent tonic to calm you down. Hyperacidity is supposedly controlled with Gulkand and also, if you are suffering from constipation, you are going to find your digestive system functioning better with this Rose jam.

The best thing I like about Gulkand is that once it is made, it is going to last for years and years. One of my relatives made it with honey, but I guess that to be overkill. After all, I am putting sugar in it, am I not. However, if you have plenty of honey around, you can make it with honey. But that is going to make it even more powerful. That means you are just going to be eating half a teaspoon, three times a day. This antioxidant is a mild laxative, and that is why it will keep your system clear and healthy.

How to collect wild rose petals – if you find red rose petals

growing in the wild, how lucky you are. This is going to have more percentage of essential oils, especially if you have Rosa Damascena around. Somehow, I do not find cultivated rose hybrids to have such a great amount of required essential oils.

Make sure that the rose petals which you collect are pesticide free by washing them thoroughly. Also get rid of the insects and dust. I normally dump them in a bucket full of water, swish them around and then strain the petals through a sieve under running water.

The sugar which you are going to use can be pounded with the petals, to make the jam making process easier. That is how they used to do it in ancient times. You may also use crystallized sugar, but that is going to make it sickly sweet. The sugar amount is going to be exactly that much as the petals. So 2 cups of petals means 2 cups of sugar. But as I am making a number of bottles, I collect about 4 cups of petals.

Gulkand is normally made in the summer. And it is going to be a slow cooking of the petals and the sugar in the sun in wide mouthed glass jars. Gulkand is definitely not made in plastic utensils. It seems the Empress NoorJahan promoted the making of rose jam in Mogul aristocratic circles, but then, we already know her historically has the lady who discovered rose oil through condensation.

Place the rose petals directly in the jars, in alternate layers. Alternating with the rose petals are going to be sugar layers. Do not fill the jar to the brim. Now, cover tightly and place out in the sun. The moisture is going to cook the jam into a jammy consistency. Give the bottle a really good shake occasionally so that the jam gets a good chance to settle down well. Your long-lasting Gulkand is going to be cooked in 2 to 3 months, in the summer. Enjoy.

 Children are fed a spoonful of Gulkand with Chyavanprash in summer, and only Chyavanprash in winter.

The Natural Cure For Sugar Diabetes

Gooseberry juice is considered to be a godsend for diabetics. Of course, diabetes can also be cured by drinking the juice of one bitter gourd twice a day, but here I am telling you of how to make sure diabetes is cured effectively.

Make up a share of equal quantities of these three juices –

One tablespoon full of Amla juice, juice of Eugenia jambolana leaves (*Jamun- which the world has discovered thanks to Oprah Winfrey,also known as Acai*) and Aeglemarmelos leaves (*bilva- the "Bel" tree*) crushed together and drunk two times a day reduces sugar in diabetic cases.

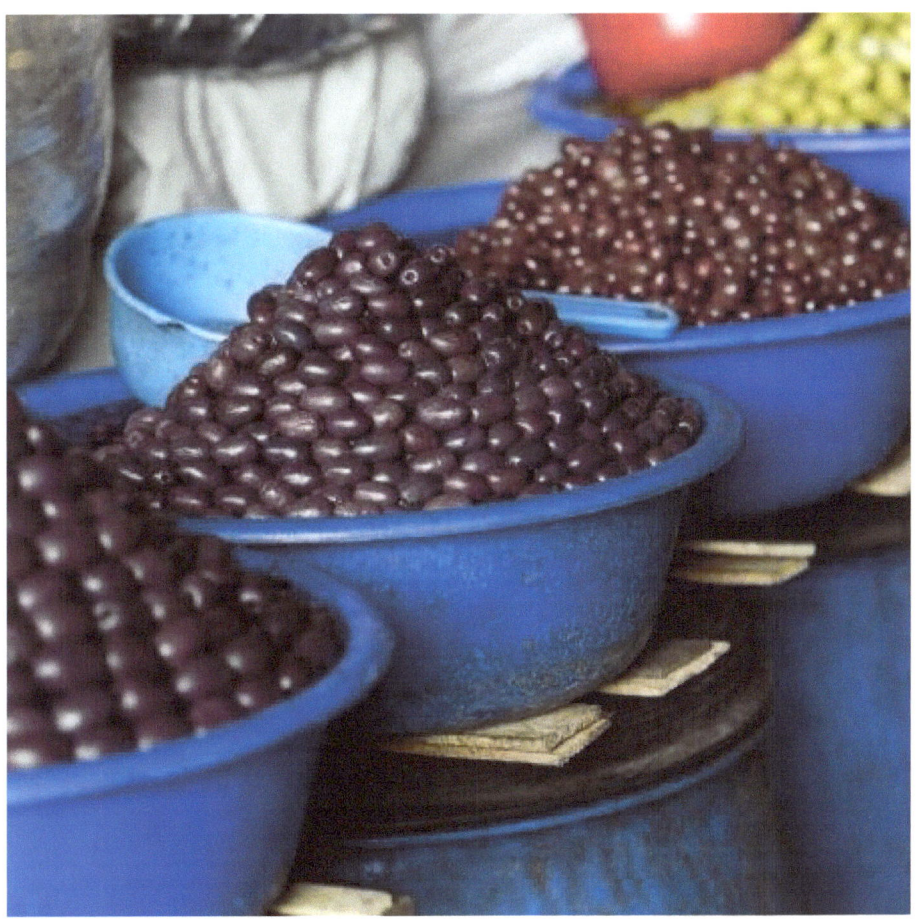

Acai is very popular in South America as well as in the East.

I am glad to note that medical Associations in America are finally finding out the efficacy of this ancient recipe. I feel good!

Talking about gooseberry juice and bitter gourd juice. I remember an instance, when I was working with a really democratic company, where trainers, administrators, staff, and faculty members sat together with the

CEO every afternoon and had lunch together. This gentleman suffered from diabetes.

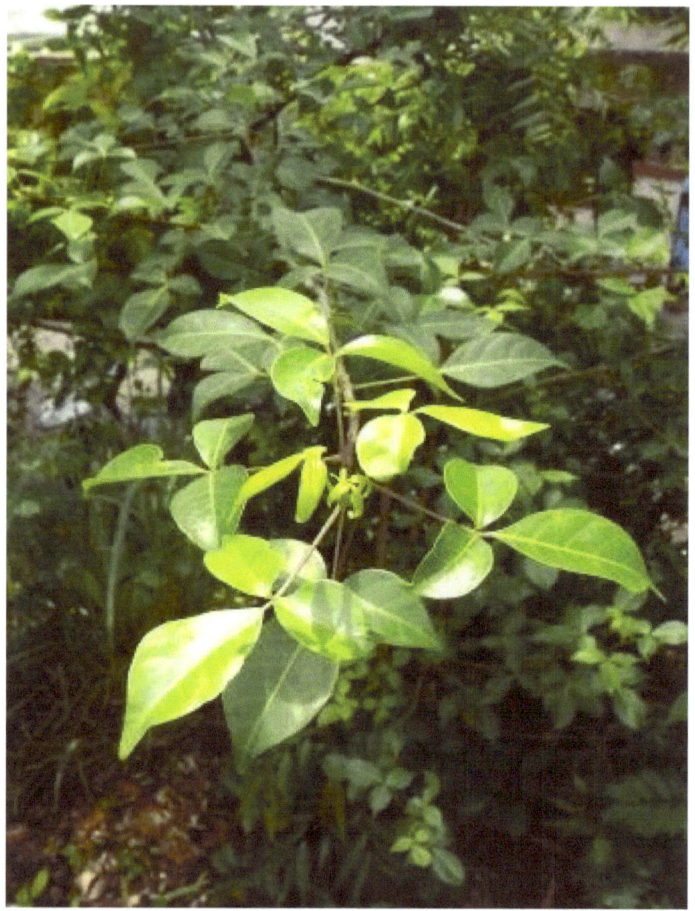

Bel leaves. The fruit of this tree is called stone apple.

His wife, who was very particular about his diet made sure that his lunch was brought piping hot in a lunchbox to the office by the servant every afternoon. It was very pleasant to laugh at him good-naturedly, especially when he used to regularly say", oh, no, not that bitter gourd juice again," and the servant telling him patiently that as long as he was suffering from diabetes, he would have to drink that juice, so there.

The time-tested rites of acception of a new colleague was a glass of this amazingly delicious looking, but oh so bitter juice, in a "toast" from new colleagues and friends in welcome – lifting up their glasses of water or lemon juice – and an admonition of "Drink up to a long, happy Association together," by the CEO, while the rest of the team tried their utmost to maintain serious faces and supposedly careless miens.

On that special day of acceptance and initiation, I got a humdinger juice mixture to my plate and portion. It was bitter gourd juice along with gooseberry juice- a really mouth puckering mixture.

So, under the avid and expectant gaze of my new colleagues, I emptied out the glass in one long gulping session. Then I licked my chops,(rather rude for a well brought up lady) contemplated the ceiling pensively and said, "Hmmmm, very nice. What is that? "

Pin drop silence. After that, our CEO, -a really nice ex- officer and gentleman- roared in best parade ground style, "So you like that, do you, Andy? You would like some more, would you now? Well, you can finish the whole lot today with my good wishes!!! It is just one flask full."

The flask was a 1.5 L one.

The lunch ended with roars of laughter at my absolutely dismayed, open mouthed and horrified look.

It did not quite end there.

In the East, long-term loyal and faithful retainers and servants consider it their prerogative to treat their masters like babies who need to be coddled and admonished for their own benefit and good!

The end result was that my CEO, often used to complain, "Thanks to you, the servant has set you up as an example by saying "*Saheb ji* (literally master sir), Andy Ma'am found that very tasty, so why are you acting like a baby and not drinking up all the juice? Now finish it, otherwise *memsaheb ji* (literally- Madam sir) will have my and your blood for breakfast." What is wrong with your taste buds, Andy? "With a look reminiscent of unspoken "weird, weird, weird human specimen."

And I used to grin sheepishly. Of course, I did not admit to him, that, having lived in the South of India, I had got used to plenty of sour, bitter and astringent drinks and dishes since childhood!

So if you are taking this juice, remember not to take more than one small glass of bitter gourd juice, with 3 tablespoons full of gooseberry juice.

Gooseberry for Increasing Brainpower

Now one wonders why students were given Chyavanprash since ancient times? That is because it is proven that brain workers would be greatly benefited if they ate gooseberries, thus increasing their brainpower.

It also increases your power of concentration, as well as improves your memory.

We were also given one spoon full of gooseberry juice, with two spoons full of honey, first thing in the morning as children. The idea was that if there was any lack of brain growth and intellectual power from the ages of one to nine, that would immediately be stimulated by the gooseberries.

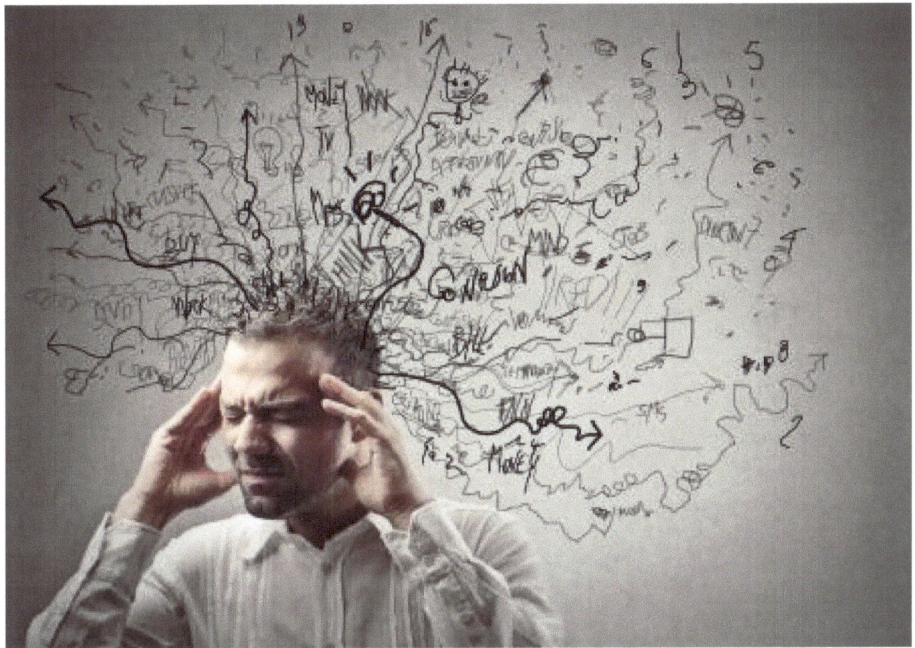

Too much stress and exertion being put on your brain? Try adding gooseberry to your diet.

Preventing Excessive Thirst and Prickly Heat

It is usual for us to feel thirsty in the summer or when the body is dehydrated, but sometimes you may feel that your thirst is not slaked even after drinking plenty of glasses of fresh fruit juice or water you find your mouth getting dry, after 10 minutes. In such a case, take 50 g dried gooseberries. Put drinking water in a utensil. Allow the gooseberries to soak in this liquid.

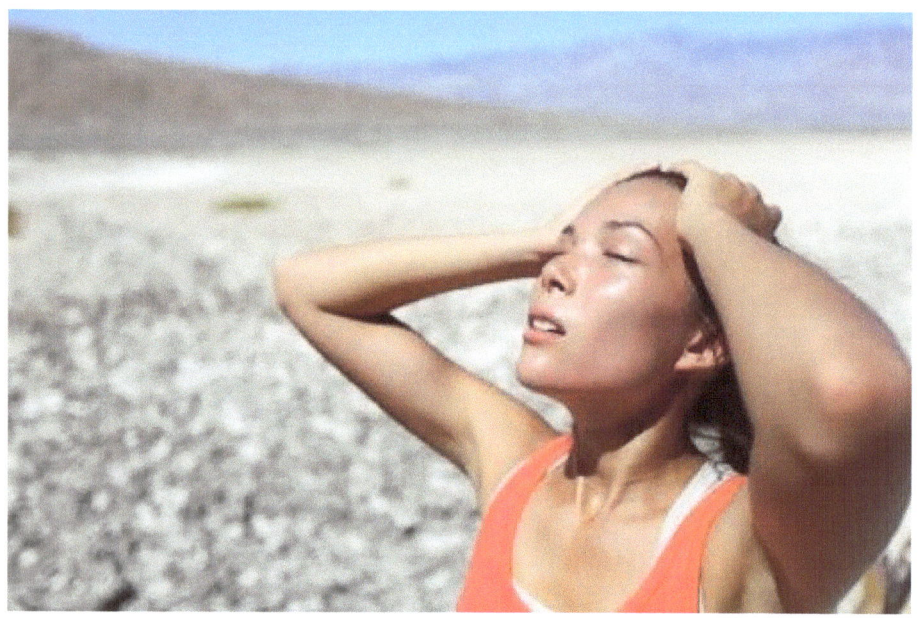

Do not ever allow yourself to reach this condition, ever, especially in the summer.

Whenever you feel thirsty throughout the day, have a glass full of gooseberry water. This is going to get rid of any electrolyte and mineral deficiency in your body, while keeping you healthy and your system toned and toxin free.

This also takes care of any prickly heat problem, which may crop up in the summer. If you keep drinking fresh lemon juice. Also, the summer, you are definitely never going to suffer from prickly heat.

Getting Rid of Cough

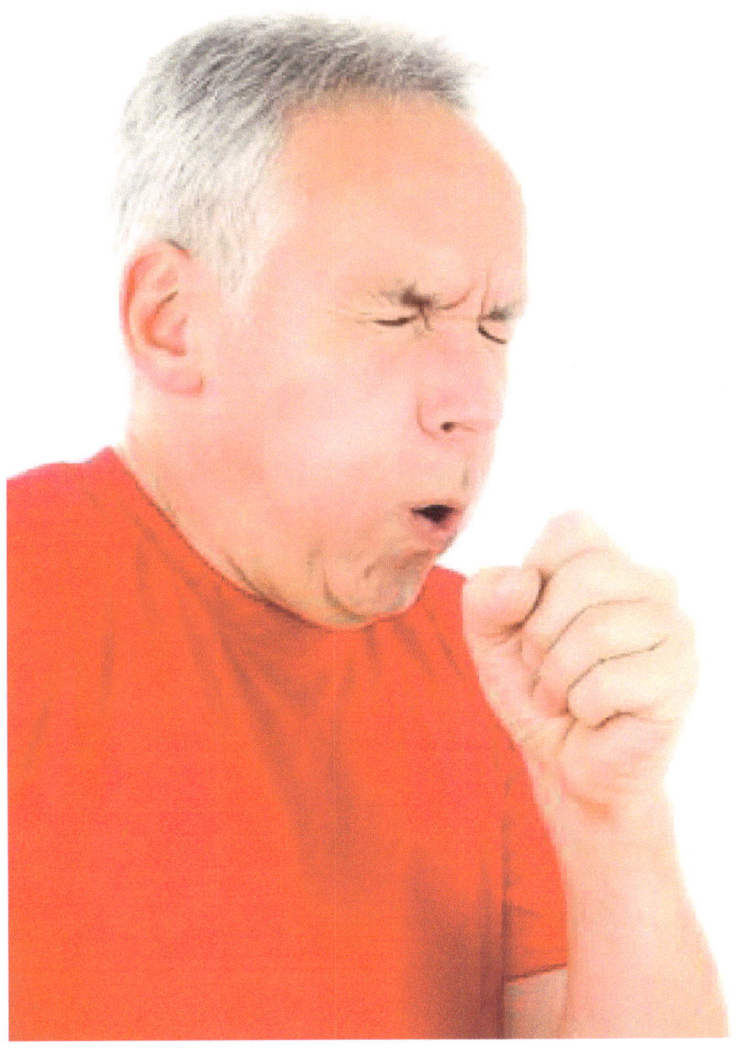

Take 20 g of powdered gooseberries. Drink with hot milk twice a day. You may want to add a little honey to the milk.

Hoarse Throat

Mix 1 teaspoon of powdered gooseberry with half a teaspoonful of honey and a little bit of licorice. Lick this mixture three times a day until your throat is cleared.

Curing Migraine

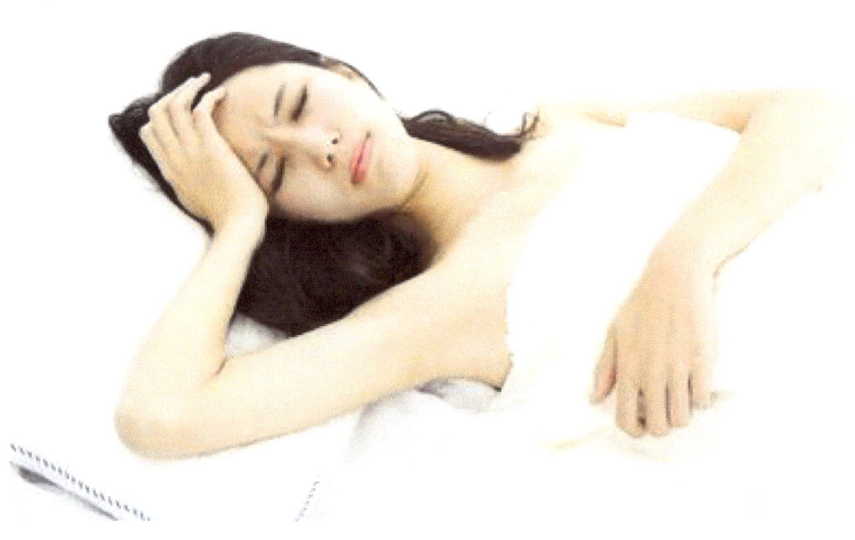

This cure was used to cure headaches and migraine, since ancient times, when there were no Migril or Vasograin tablets around. Make a paste of powdered gooseberry, with rosewater. Apply this paste all over your forehead. This is going to help cure your headache or migraine attack.

How Useful Is Gooseberry with Honey

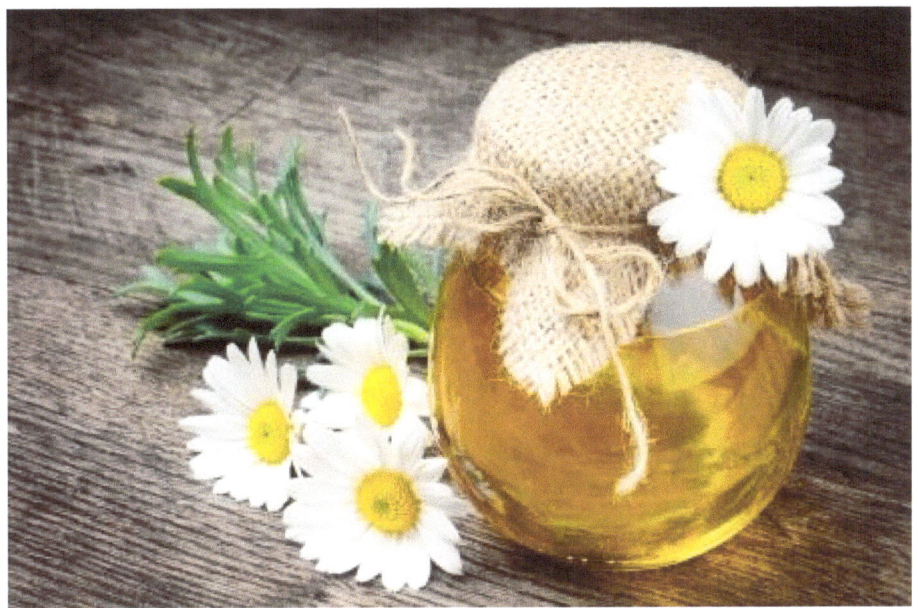

The gooseberry honey combination is extremely useful in a number of ailments. You just have to mix half a teaspoonful of gooseberry powder with half a teaspoonful of honey and drink it up with warm milk twice a day, to cure chronic cases of this entry, nausea, premature whitening of hair, hair fall, nosebleed and urinary inconsistency. For this last ailment, follow-up with two bananas.

Try This Tip
Start eating about 2 g of powdered gooseberry, with a little bit of honey, the last thing you do before you go to sleep. And then look at its multifarious and very effective health restoring benefits, after its regular use over a given period of time.

Preventing Vitamin C Deficiency

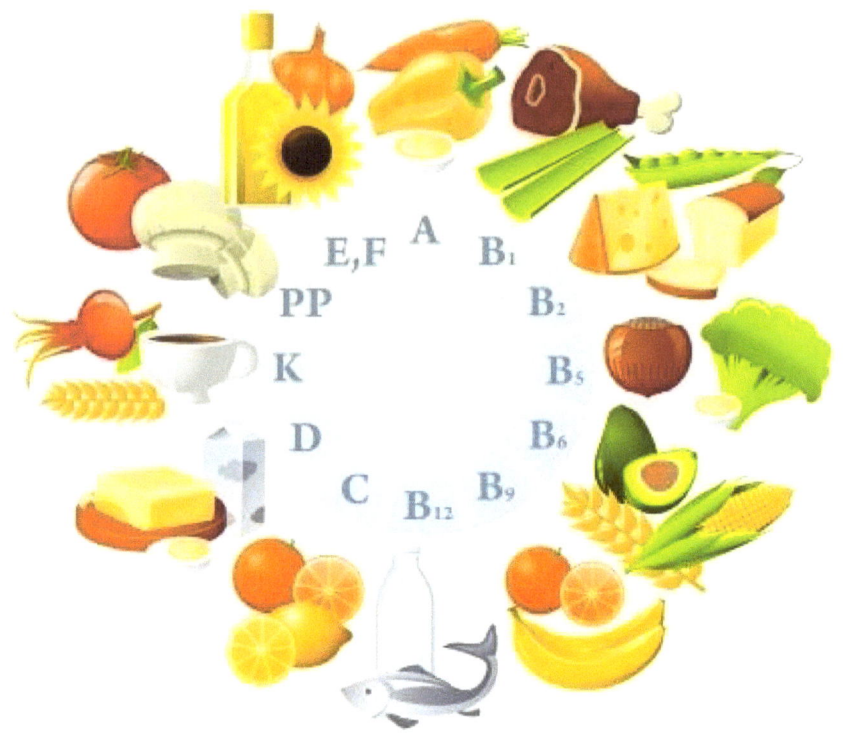

In the East, wise men advocated catching children young and feeding them with nourishing food, so that they never suffered from any sort of deficiency within the grew up. So a new born child was fed 2 grams each of honey and fresh gooseberry juice, twice a day until it reached the age of four years. When he was four, he was fed 3 g each of honey and gooseberry juice, four times a day, without fail. This prevented any vitamin deficiency.

In the same way, adults suffering from beriberi and scurvy can also be fed this remedy, until they begin to show positive results.

Liver Problems

Now this is an ancient Ayurvedic remedy, which definitely does not have any scientific backing or standing, but it was used for millenniums to cure problems in the liver. This is because the gooseberry promoted the liver's well-being.

Take 3 g of powdered gooseberry, 2.5 g each of dried ginger, black peppercorns, turmeric, and pippali.

http://www.medindia.net/alternativemedicine/pippali.asp

This last indigenous herb is also called Long pepper in English. You are going to eat its dry spike. Make up a mixture of all these ingredients. Now eat just one gram of this powder with half a teaspoonful of sugar every day.

You are going to find your liver beginning to work properly, within less than two months. I wondered whether this can be a good remedy for people suffering from cirrhosis of the liver or other liver related diseases. The village doctor who gave me this remedy assured me that he was treating a heavy drinker with this cure. Of course he had to stop drinking, in order to get his liver functioning again.

Curing Jaundice

Jaundice is normally caused when the RBC count lowers in the body. This is because the liver is not functioning properly. In the East, jaundice is normally sure to with drinking lots of sugarcane juice with lemon. So the next time you see somebody suffering from jaundice, give him 3 g of gooseberry juice in a glass of buttermilk, once a day until he is cured. This is going to tone up the liver.

Gooseberries for Beauty

Gooseberries are considered to be the best way in which you can promote hair growth. The seeds are crushed to make Gooseberry oil, which is then added to coconut oil. This oil massaged in the scalp, before a shampoo is considered to be an excellent promoter of hair growth.

Suffering from Skin Ailments?

This remedy is normally used by adolescent girls in the East, to make sure that they do not suffer from any puberty related skin problems like pimples, blemishes, blackheads, etc.. Powder, some dried gooseberries and soak them overnight in water. Early in the morning, wash your face with that water. This is going to prevent or get rid of pimples, and clear of your skin. You are also going to find your skin glowing.

Making a Gooseberry Skincare Cream

I learned this recipe in a village where they still use coals and clay pots for cooking. Children suffering from skin diseases are normally treated with this skincare cream. You may not make this recipe, unless you have coals, but this is a traditional way in which dried gooseberries were burnt in charcoal fires. Put the dried gooseberries in a small clay utensil. Seal its mouth with a mud seal. Now apply a paste of mud all over that container. Put the container in the coals, cook your dinner in the fire, and by the time your dinner is prepared – about one hour, you are going to find that the dried gooseberries have been burnt to a crisp charcoal.

Now, grind these burnt pieces and mix them with any oil, coconut oil, mustard oil or sesame oil. You are now going to get an ointment which you can apply on any infected area on the skin. Firstly, make sure that the patient regularly washes that affected area with neem leaves.. This neem water is going to be made up of 25 to 30 fresh neem leaves steeped in water for 20 minutes. The patient is going to have a bath with this neem water. After that, apply the gooseberry cream on the affected areas.

 It does not matter whether the skin ailment is dry – itching – or infected – pimples –. A regular use of this skin cream is going to help cure your skin properly.

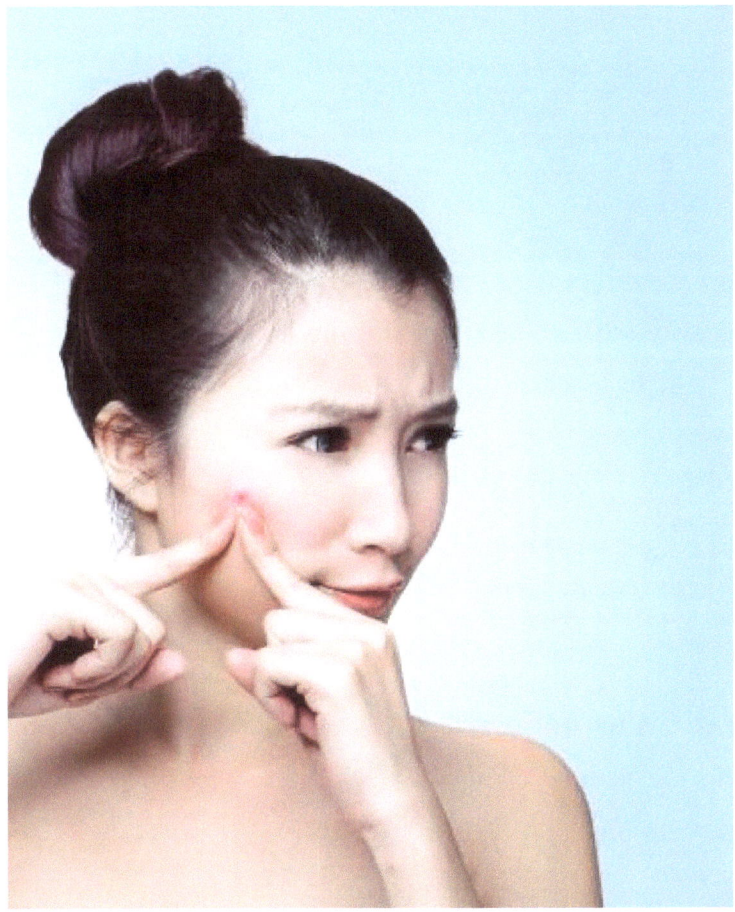

No squeezing, please! That will spread the infection.

Hair Loss Recipe

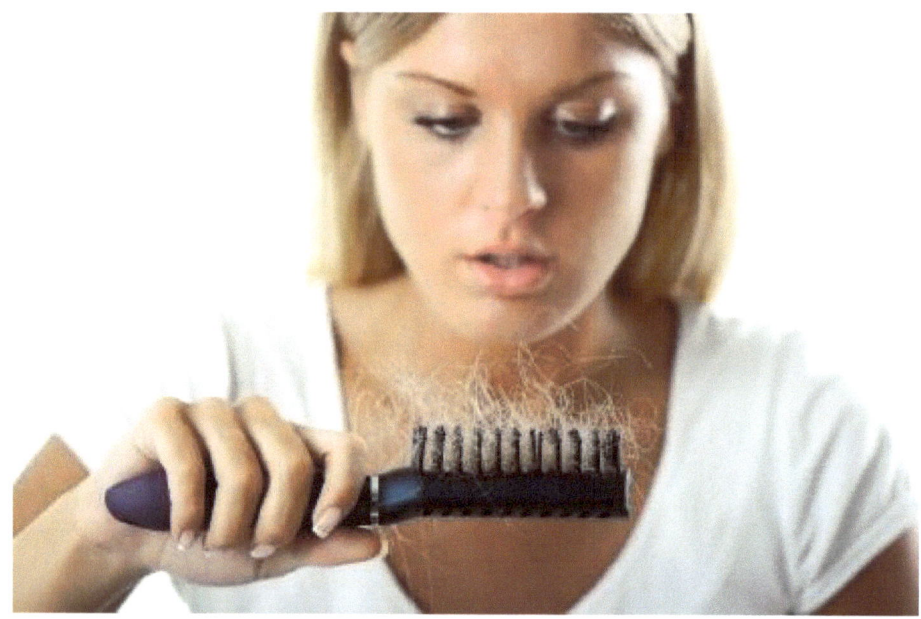

If this is distressing and a regular feature every day, make sure that you have a healthy diet. Also go in for a checkup.

Make a mixture of Amla (Emblica officianalis powder) in freshly squeezed lime juice. Massage your scalp with this mixture. Not only will it prevent hair from growing gray, but it will ensure that hair loss is also drastically reduced.

Natural Conditioners for the Hair

This is the best natural conditioning recipe, for your hair, to remove all the frizz and dryness.

Two tablespoons yoghurt

50 g papaya

Two eggs

Two tablespoons honey

Mix up all these ingredients well and apply them onto your hair. Leave this pack on your hair for about an hour. After that, shampoo your hair and massage the scalp with warm coconut or olive oil.

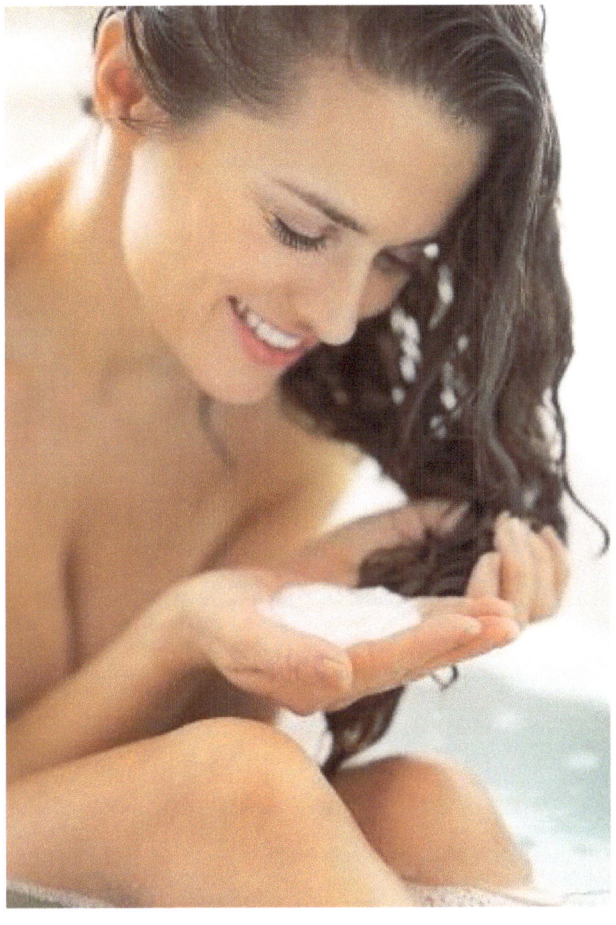

The best hair conditioner is, of course, coconut oil!

Anybody who imagines that the regular application of oil can darken your hair roots is deluding himself. Any beauty product which tries to beguile you into buying oil which will turn your hair black again is cheating you. These marketing gimmicks are worthless, but then you should remember that the natural color of your hair is natural, anything applied onto it is a superficial coating which makes it look soft, and lustrous.

Now the natural Eastern way of darkening your hair and making it long, soft, clean, dark and lustrous is done by our ancient time tested herbal remedy called the soap nut formula. We did not use any shampoos except soap nuts which we also used as a safe and mild detergent to wash our warm clothes, through the centuries.

If you do not have dark hair, do not make the shampoo in the iron pot.

Traditional Natural Shampoo

Ingredients in the Shampoo

The Indian soap nut Ritha -Sapindus Mukorosse- is the best natural shampoo because the saponins present in their outer shell makes a foamy lather when it comes in contact with water. A soap nut has a hard black inner seed which we normally add to garden compost.

Shikakai is the dried pods of a native plant. These are shelled and the outer shell used in the shampoos.

Emblica officinalis (gooseberry- Amla)- dried powdered gooseberry is one of the most powerful herbal remedies used in Indian natural medicine. At the moment, I am using gooseberries to prepare a shampoo

Eclipta alba (Bhringraj)—this is a powdered herb which is an essential part of keeping your hair long and healthy.

http://en.wikipedia.org/wiki/Eclipta_alba

Jabakusum- Hibiscus Rosa sinensis—the attractive flowers of the ordinary Hibiscus are very valuable as additives in the natural hair conditioner and shampoo. You can either use fresh flowers or dried flowers to put into your iron cauldron in which you are going to brew this powerful shampoo. You can also use Arnica to add more power to the brew.

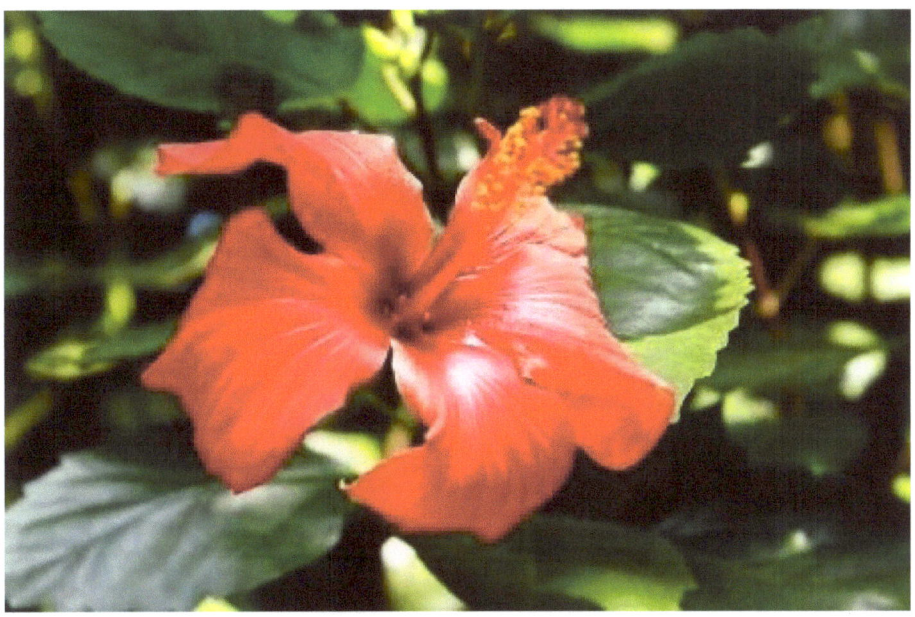

Dried Hibiscus – China rose – petals are excellent for your hair.

Bubble bubble, a little bit of trouble, brunettes prepare an iron vessel. Blondes and auburn haired folk, get out any ordinary kitchen container.

To this container add hundred grams each of dried Bhringraj, Amla, Shikakai,Ritha , hibiscus flowers and Arnica and using your favorite good Karma incantation, *"I am making you with lots of care,hair there and everywhere, give me long, lovely, soft, ad standard hair."*

Bring the mixture to a boil. Let it cool down and then apply this lotion/ potion to your hair with a brush. This is the best hair softener and after a couple of hours you can wash it out with a **soapnut solution**.

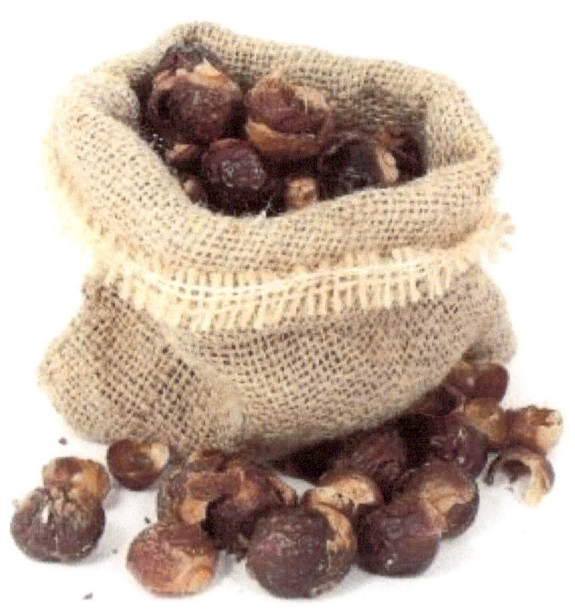

Dried soap nuts also known as washing – nuts

That is rather easy to make. 10 peeled soap nuts in half litres of water. Bring to a boil, let the soapy mixture cool down and then use this instead of a chemical shampoo. It is soft enough for your hands and hair.

We also use the soapnut as a detergent in our washing machines. We put a couple of soap nuts in the wash bag instead of a detergent and let the saponins do the work. The clothes turn out clean and soft.

I remember my paternal grandmother, boiling our winter clothes in a huge vessel with soap nuts and neem leaves with a miniscule touch of copper sulfate before packing them away in their protective coverings. She also put in a couple of handfuls of dried neem leaves in the boxes to discourage the silverfish and moths, because nobody really knew about napthalene balls in her village.

The best Diet for long and lovely hair is of course plenty of proteins, eggs, fish, and green vegetables. The use of an oil to massage the scalp is useful enough to stimulate and encourage the hair follicles to grow.

Best Natural Rinse after a Shampoo

If you have healthy and normal hair, add some dried marigold flower petals, and one tablespoon of tea to water and let the mixture boil for five minutes. Strain it and pour it over your hair after the shampoo to give your hair shine and bounce. Who needs ph graded expensive rinses?

I even put Marigold and hibiscus flowers in my shampoo of amla, retha bhringraj and shikakai.

These ingredients are peeled , and then placed in an iron vessel. Then, the liquid is boiled to make a black soapy shampoo. Forget about hair fall, forget about hair dye. This is the secret of those lovely dark tresses of the ladies of the East, Bengal predominantly. They call hibiscus Jabakusum. Of course it sounds a very messy and time-consuming procedure, but if you consider yourself self-worth it, it is worth it.

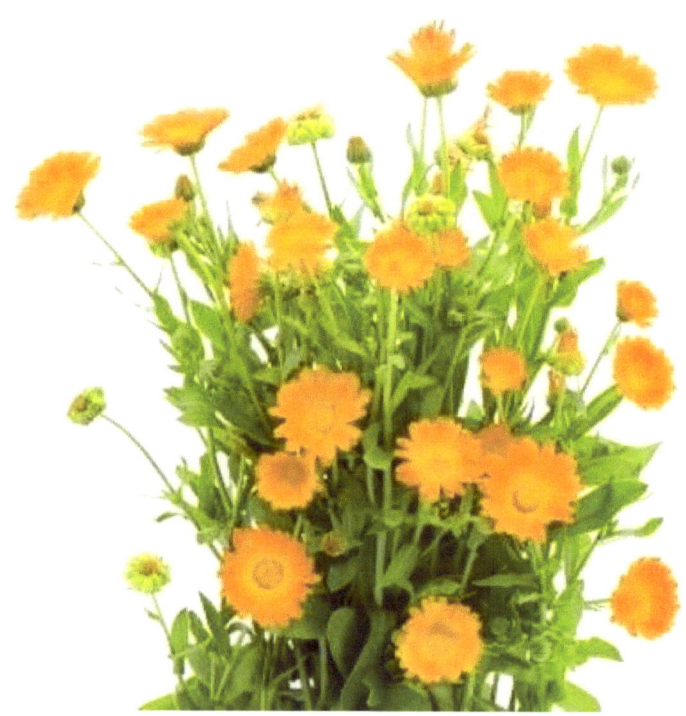

Dried calendula – Marigold petals are excellent for your hair

Here is the rosewater recipe –

Rosewater is normally available in markets at exorbitant prices, but in India, anybody with access to the red rose - Rosa Damascena, - used in India and Iran or Rosa Centifolia which is used in Bulgaria, and Germany-and a little bit of time enjoys making Rosewater at home. This Rosewater is used in cosmetics, as well as in cookery to impart the flavor of the Rose to your meal or to your skin.

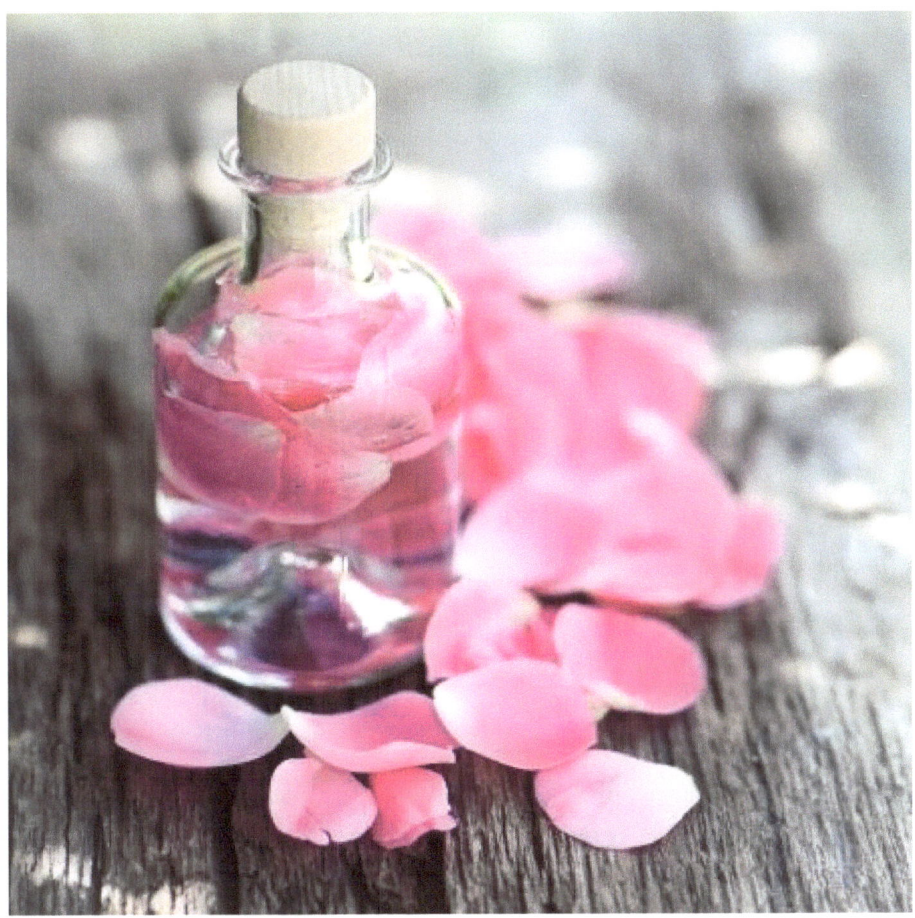

How to make Rose water (Gulab Jal)

Ingredients needed- 1 Cup Rose petals - 12 to 14 flowers.

2 cups water

Lots of ice.

A huge cooking pan - pan number one - with lid in which another pan - pan number two - can be placed comfortably.

Rosewater is just a matter of distillation. Put a wire stand in pan number one, on which you are going to stand the other pan number two. The condensed Rosewater is going to fall into pan number two.

Place the petals at the bottom of the pan number one. Now, cover the petals with water. Place pan number two on the wire stand. Now take the lid and place it upside down on pan number one, thus effectively covering the Rose petals, pan number two and the water. The Rose water is going to condense when you place the blocks and chunks of ice on the inverted lid.

You are going to have a cupful of precious distilled Rosewater, after 25 minutes of slow steaming of the Rose petals.

Precautions - remember to have enough of water to cover the Rose petals. Also, it should not be of such a large quantity, that it displaces the wire stand.

This cooled water is now pure Rosewater. Place it in a sterilized glass bottle. Use it to your heart's content. You may see a little bit of oil swimming over the surface of the water. This is Rose oil, and is even more precious. So if you used lots of petals in a larger pan, you may find even more Rose oil.

This method is for all those people who use a pressure cooker while cooking food. In fact, it is a common way to cook food in Asian kitchens, instead of using the microwave.

You would need water, petals, a pressure cooker and a long thin pipe which it does not melt, when subjected to heat.

Put the water and the petals in the pressure cooker and cover it. Now cover the thin pipe with wet cloth in order to keep it cool. Attach this pipe on the lid of the pressure cooker where you normally attach the weight. Allow the petals to cook slowly, they seem to build up, go through the cooled pipe and collect in a utensil. I tried this way too, but I find the ice on the lid one easier!

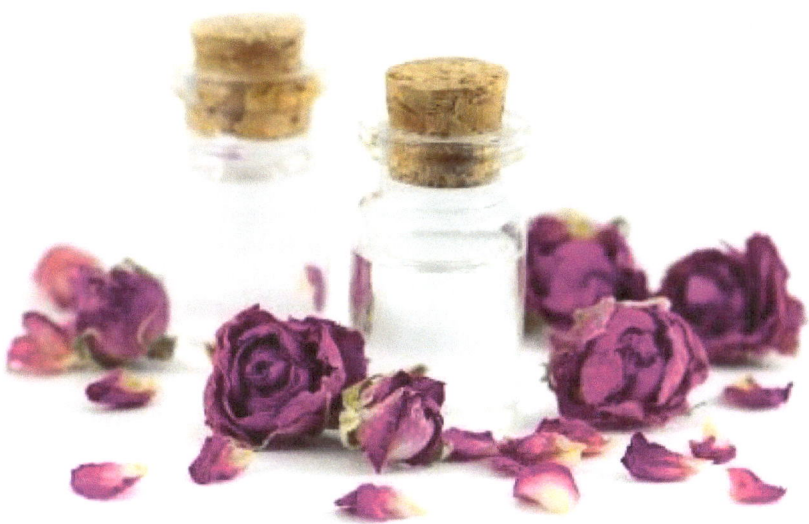

Rose essential oil is an important and very precious side product, when you make rosewater. 20,000 rose petals make 1 g of essential oil

So now that you know all about how to make rosewater, you can use it to beautify your skin, especially as an additive to a facemask in which you have put powdered gooseberries.

Natural Hair Dye

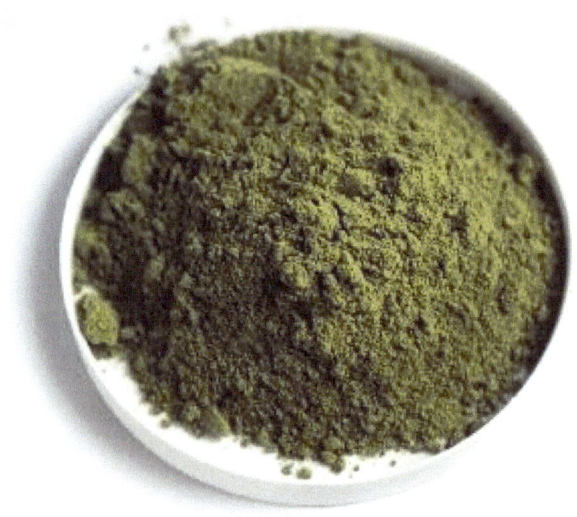

Henna is a natural hair dye and conditioner, but it leaves your hair auburn.

Now I am going to tell you all about a natural dye, to darken your hair. Do not use the chemical-based hair dies available in the market, because they cause skin problems like itchiness of the skin and possible eczema.

Take half a cup of dried gooseberries, and allow them to soak overnight in water. In the morning, wash your hair with the gooseberries pulped in that water. Do not use any other shampoo. This is going to darken your hair, if you use it two times a week regularly.

It is a well-known fact in the East, that gooseberries are the best way in which you can keep your hair black. That is because they darken the hair from the roots. So if you are suffering from white hair, try this remedy. You are going to be surprised to see dark hair growth. Also remember to add fresh gooseberries to your diet from today.

The dye is going to be made when you decide to dye. Seriously speaking, even though I am in my late 40s, there is no question of my dyeing my hair if I ever suffer from premature grayness. That is because a regular gooseberry diet is going to make sure that they do not grow gray in the first place. However, if you have already reached the stage when you have a head full of gray hair, use this dye to darken your hair naturally and to promote dark cell growth from the roots.

Take 1 kg of gooseberry juice, 1 kg of desi ghee, [I will be telling you the recipe of how to make this clarified butter, after I give you this dyeing remedy.], 250 g of the caress. Heat them all together on low heat. When the water dries up and you find just an oily residue, you need to filter it, and put it in a glass bottle. This is now an extremely powerful oil. Use it as a hair dye.

You are going to see your hair growing black within the week. I have seen this work on a lady in her 70s, and her friends asked her, how her hair had turned black between one meeting to the other. She showed them the newly growing black roots, to their great amazement and wonder. So you does not mean that the moment you reach your 50s and 60s, you have to suffer from the distinguished looking grayness of hair.

Also, she told me that this oil seems to have rejuvenated her brain, because she is learning a new language, now. And she is beating her much younger classmates hands-down with her memory retentive power to the great astonishment of her instructor.

My Own Shampoo

In the same way, if you use my shampoo every day on your hair to keep your hair black and silky, it is going to be extremely beneficial. Just add the juice of half a lemon to your washing water. Then add a spoonful of powdered gooseberry to this water. Wash your hair in it every day. This is going to darken your hair naturally and keep it soft and silky because of the lemon conditioner.

Hair Darkener

Here is another hair darkener , which I saw demonstrated of a weekend a couple of years ago. Take 10 dried gooseberries. Now make into a paste with 15 to 20 leaves of Henna and Neem. Grind them in milk into a paste, apply on the areas which are graying, and let it dry in an hour. After that, wash your hair with my shampoo given above. [Lemon and gooseberry powder.] Do this twice a week. Believe it or not, your hair will start to darken within two months, depending on their stage of grayness.

How to Make Gooseberry Hair Oil

Remember to apply this hair oil, on your freshly shampoo-ed hair only after your hair are completely dry and tangle free.

Take 4 kg of raw gooseberries. You may want to cut or chop them for faster absorption of oil. Now add them in 4 kg of sesame oil. Place the oil in a glass bottle and in the sun for about 15 days. Now this powerful filtered oil is considered to be an integral part of an Indian's haircare products. If you go buying it in the market, you are going to see it selling at exorbitant prices. But here I am, giving you the recipe. So make your own hair darkening oil right at home.

Why 4 kg of gooseberries, you may say? Well, that is because everyone in the neighborhood is going to ask you for your special homemade oil. So it is better to get this made in large quantities in first go itself.

Taking Care of Your Teeth

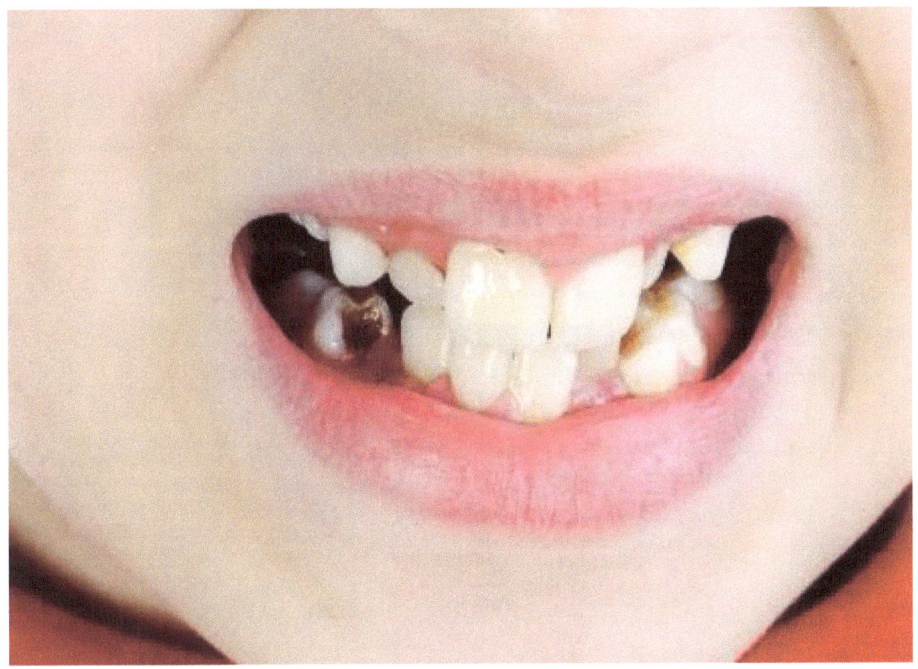

This dental problem would have been avoided if he had eaten more gooseberries…

I was surprised to hear that dentists mostly do not advise their patients not to drink cold liquids, after they have hot liquids. This is the easiest way in which you can cause harm to your teeth. So here are some easy tips, with which you can preserve your teeth, thanks to gooseberries.

Firstly, remember to rinse your mouth out with water, after you have eaten anything, including snacks, meals, and other chewable items. In the East, the tradition is to fill your mouth up with water, brush your teeth with a finger to get rid of any lurking food particles and spit out the water. After that, you gargle water to clear your throat. Remember to spit it out too! We learned these habits since early childhood until they became second nature. And that is why we do not bother much about dentists now.

Dental problems like caries and rotting teeth can definitely be prevented by eating fresh gooseberries every day. I believe, that was the reason why a childhood full of gooseberries kept our teeth sparkling clean, just like apples did.

 If it is not the season of the gooseberry, you can soak 4 pieces of dried gooseberries in water overnight, and chew them in the morning.

Grandmothers in Asia relieve teething problems in their kids by rubbing the gums with gooseberry juice. Also, you can make up the gripe water being sold in the market by adding 3 teaspoons full of Bishops Weed [Lovage] in water, boiling it, cooling it, and giving a teaspoonful to baby, whenever he feels uneasy.

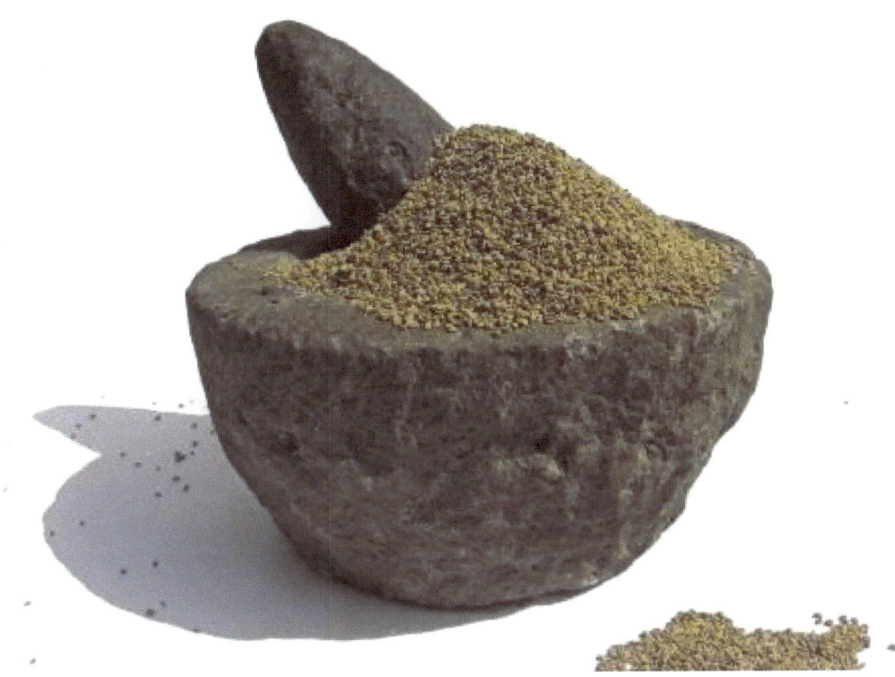

Bishops Weed ready for grinding in a traditional stone pestle and mortar.

Pyorreah

I normally use mustard oil and salt to keep my guns healthy, but here is another remedy, which is a guaranteed cure for even chronic cases of rotting and bleeding gums. Add one teaspoonful of gooseberry powder to 10 teaspoonfuls of mustard oil. Now slowly and gently massage your bleeding gums with this mixture twice a day. The mustard oil is going to cure your bleeding gums. The gooseberry is going to prevent any sort of infection spreading in your mouth.

Shaking teeth

Try eating fresh gooseberries every day. Chewing these gooseberries are going to firm your teeth in their respective places. That is because the vitamin C helps your teeth grow stronger.

You can also try this remedy. Boil some pieces of gooseberry in water, and allow to cool to bearable hot. Now gargle with this hot water, and massage your teeth gently. After that, spit out the hot water and gargle with a mouthful of cold water. Do this five times. This hot cold gargle has to be done once a day, until your teeth regain their firmness.

Gooseberries in Traditional Cooking

Apart from using gooseberries in pies, "fools" and other traditional British cooking, gooseberries are also used in making chutneys and pickles.

Gooseberry Chutney

Traditional Gooseberry chutney is normally made by cutting up unripe gooseberries and mixing them with rock salt, ginger, pepper, garlic and onions, according to taste. Grind them together. If you want to preserve this chutney, put in more salt before bottling. If you want to eat it fresh, you may want to add red chilies/green chilies to make it spicier.

I give it the sweet, sour taste by adding one spoon full of molasses before grinding. So if you are suffering from any tummy problems, you may want to have a spoonful of this delicious chutney, with your meals. This is going to increase your appetite as well as make sure that you have a healthy digestive system.

Sometimes, I also add a little bit of mint and coriander [cilantro] leaves to this chutney. This is excellent with snacks and with finger foods.

Traditional Gooseberry jam

I am sure your grandma told you that gooseberries were excellent fruit to make into jams. This is the traditional Gooseberry jam recipe used in the East. Did you know that Indian royalty used to eat this gooseberry jam for breakfast with a thin layer of silver foil over it. This foil is made up of beating real silver into thin sheets, and is called "vark". It is considered to be the epitome of exotic, luxurious and rich living.

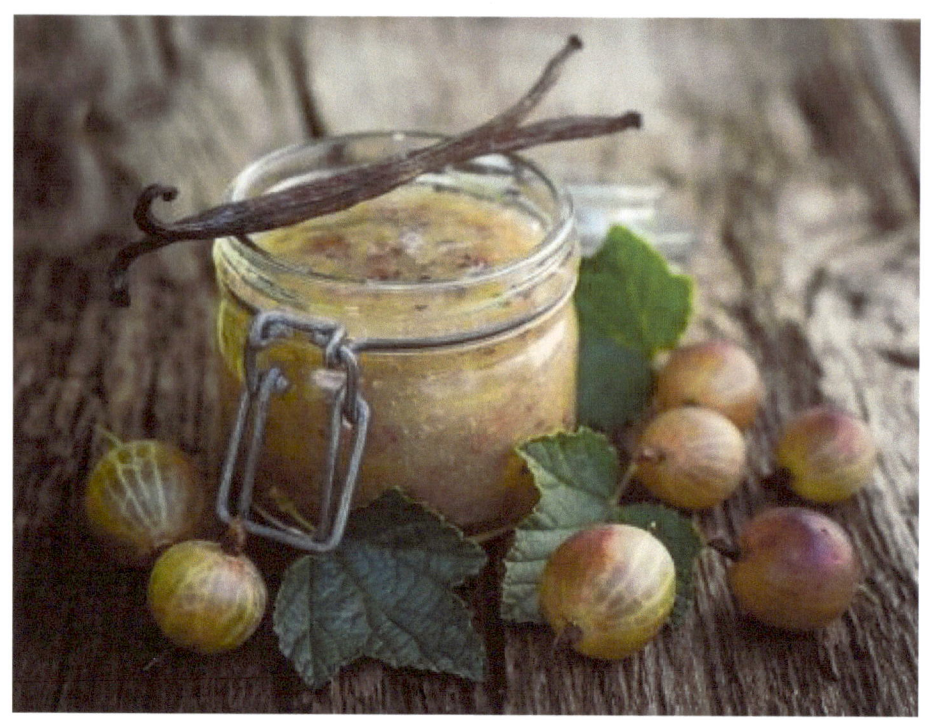

Gooseberry jam eaten for breakfast

Traditional jam is made up of collecting ripe gooseberries and then washing them thoroughly to remove pesticides and traces of dirt. After that, these gooseberries are pierced with a fork and left for 24 hours in lime (choona) water. This is a time taking process, which will need you to make fresh sugar syrups at least three – four times.

When you are ready to make the jam, take the fruit out from the lime water and wash in running water to get rid of any vestiges of the lime. You may want to cut it in small pieces, now. Or you may want to leave the fruit intact, but that means that you are also going to have the seeds in the jam.

Now make a thick syrup of sugar and put the gooseberries in it. Place in a glass bottle. The next day, remove the gooseberries from the syrup, and make some more fresh syrup. I would suggest syrup made of 1 cup sugar. Add the gooseberries to the old and the fresh syrup. Repeat this making of the new syrup procedure four days running. After that place the glass container in the sun, and allow the syrup to be absorbed in the fruit. One teaspoonful of this jam for breakfast is much better than orange marmalade!

Traditional Gooseberry pickles

Fruit and vegetables are preserved in the East by picking or being made into jam, as soon as they are harvested.

So here is my favorite recipe for traditional gooseberry pickles in oil. Use the oil you like best. I use mustard oil, but because it is an acquired taste, you can use any sort of good cooking oil.

Half Kg gooseberry fruit pulp – seedless gooseberry flesh boiled in water for a little while, so that it turns soft, but does not turn into a formless mass.

4 tablespoonful Salt.
One teaspoonful rocksalt.
Two tablespoonfuls of dried chilies. This is going to make the pickles really hot. If you want a milder pickle, Deseed the chillies.
2 tablespoons minced garlic
1 tablespoon black pepper
1 teaspoon dried ginger powder

Spices – 2 tablespoons each of fenugreek seeds, yellow mustard seeds, coriander seeds, cumin seeds nigella and Bishops Weed. Roast the cumin and grind. Leave the rest of the seeds as they are. This makes the basic pickle spice mixture.

Spread the Gooseberry pulp on a large platter and dust with all the spices. Heat the oil until it "smokes" and lower the heat. Allow it to cool. Put the Gooseberry and the spices in a wide mouthed glass jar. Cover it with oil and place in the sun for six days. Stir once or twice daily. It is going to be ready for eating within the week.

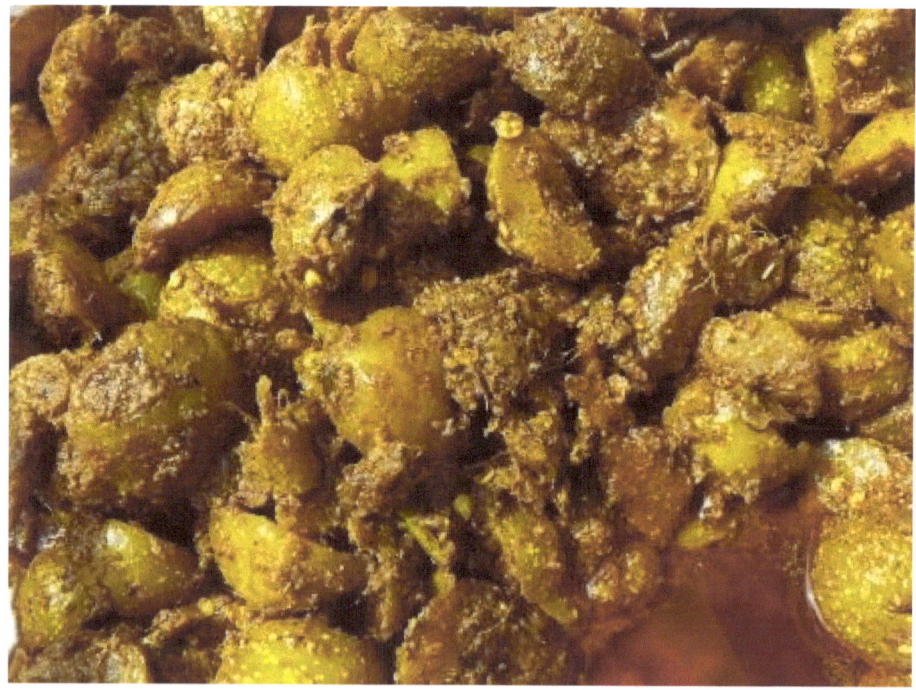

This is how it is going to look like when cooked in the sun

My friends use another way of making this pickle. They fry all the spices in oil, and then put in the Gooseberry, as if they are making something tasty for lunch. But that lunch is going to be covered with more oil, and is going to cook in the sun for a long long time. In fact, they believed that the more pickles are cooked in the sun, the better, and tastier they are in the long run.

In lieu of sunshine, you may place the glass jar in a warm dry place in your kitchen, near a source of heat. One of my friends in Canada suggested placing it near hot water pipes or the kitchen boiler. Good idea. Keep the jar dry, keep rotating it, so that the heat does not bake just one particular area, do not use the lid during the day, but cover it with a thin Muslin, but cover with lid at night. The place should be cool and dry.

The Difference between Chutneys and Pickles

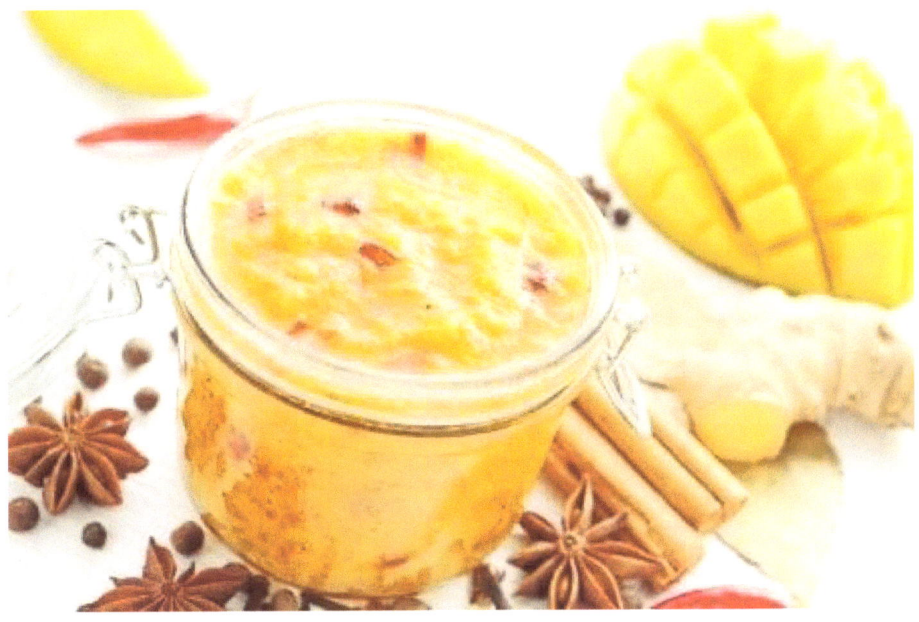

Mango chutney made of spices in vinegar

Chutneys are normally made of apple or organic vinegar, spices and sugar. Pickles are marinated in oil. The pickles can either be cooked before they are placed in oil or they can be put in raw with plenty of salt.

Traditional Eastern pickles are rarely exported to the west, because they are made for home use, by the ladies of the house, every winter. Each long-lived house has its own particular pickle recipe and tradition. On the other hand, chutneys are exported to the West and are very popular, there.

The commercial pickles that you buy in the West are made by companies, which put in preservatives and overseason the pulp. These are then passed off as traditional Eastern recipes. They are about as different from the real thing as, say, a steamed pudding is different from a delicately made soufflé.

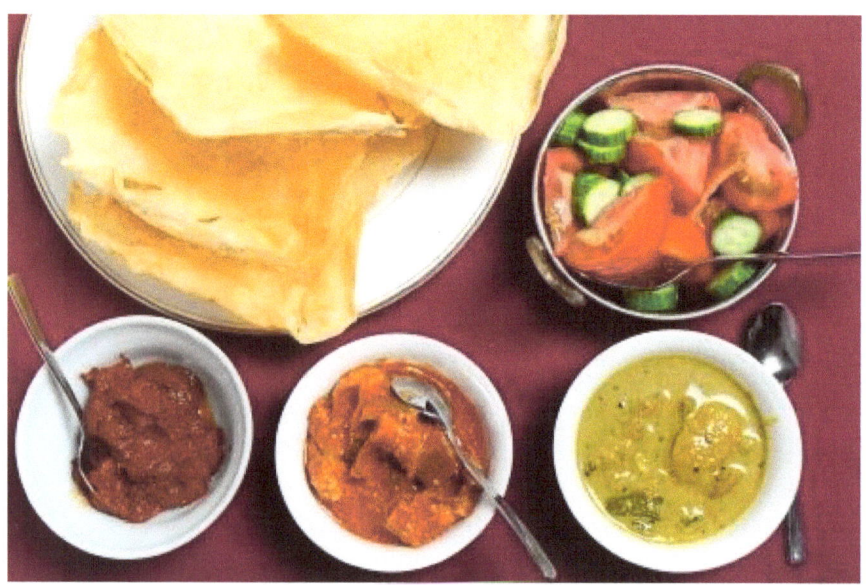

Traditional tomato, mango, and white lime pickles as accompaniments to salads and poppadoms.

Conclusion

Believe it or not, I have not managed to touch a fraction of the uses to which you can put gooseberries. That is because any researcher is going to be confused at all the remedies in which this versatile fruit plays a major role. Nevertheless, remember that gooseberries should be an integral part of your diet, whether eaten raw or in cooked form.

How to Dry Gooseberries?

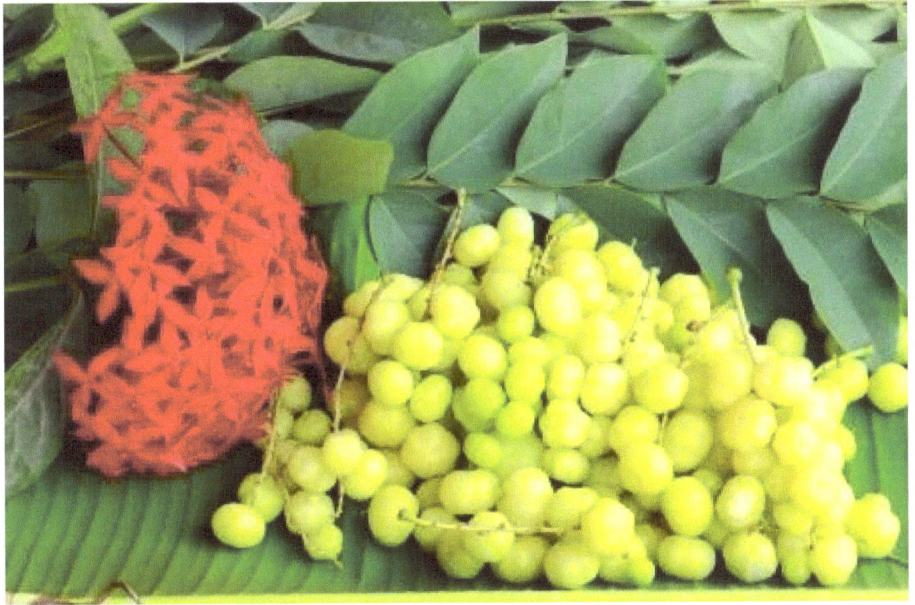

These need to be sun-dried…

You sun dry gooseberries by cutting them into small pieces, and placing them in the shade in a sunny part of your roof terrace or on your kitchen sill. The gooseberries are going to get dehydrated in 6 to 8 days. You may either keep them as they are, for soaking overnight and eating purposes, or you may powder them, depending on the use to which you want to put them.

Desi Ghee

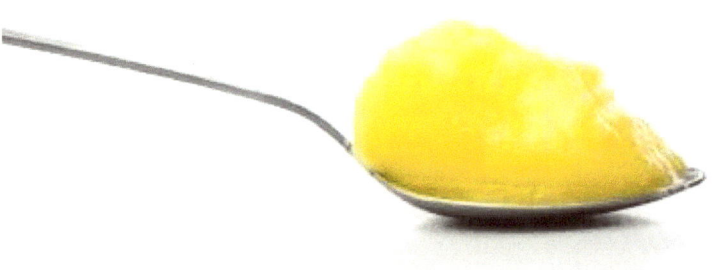

Pure clarified butter is concentrated in consistency and golden yellow in color.

One of the recipes given above spoke about Desi ghee. This is clarified butter, which is extremely concentrated and a very powerful healing agent. It is normally used in the making up of herbal medicines, because it is made of pure creamy milk butter.

Desi ghee is the concentrated form of pure butter, which is heated to reduce the butter of all the impurities as well as moisture. This concentrated butter is normally used in Eastern cuisine, for searing meat, sautéing and frying food, because they offer its higher burning point. You make this at home by taking 2 pounds of best unsalted butter and melting it in a heavy bottomed pan. Allow the butter to liquefy on low heat for about 40 minutes. Maintain this simmering point, until all of the moisture in the butter has evaporated. The impurities are going to sink to the bottom of the pan. Remember to keep stirring the butter, so that it does not burn.

Pour off the clear butter and strain it through several thicknesses of muslin cloth. This butter is going to last for about a year, if it is placed in a cool and dry place. This butter is exorbitantly expensive. So in the East, people with easy access to plenty fresh milk make it right in their kitchens for crisp delicious frying results, and adding that taste of pure butter to all their dishes.

Now that you know all about the power of the Gooseberry, take full advantage of all, it is natural benefits right now. Remember, all the natural herbs, vegetables, fruits and spices that we get out there have been placed on this earth for the benefit of mankind. So make sure that you utilize this knowledge to keep yourself fit, fine and healthy.

Live a happy and healthy life with gooseberries.

Author Bio

Dueep Jyot Singh is a Management and IT Professional who managed to gather Postgraduate qualifications in Management and English and Degrees in Science, French and Education while pursuing different enjoyable career options like being an hospital administrator, IT,SEO and HRD Database Manager/ trainer, movie scriptwriter, theatre artiste and public speaker, lecturer in French, Marketing and Advertising, ex-Editor of Hearts On Fire (now known as Solctice) Books Missouri USA, advice columnist and cartoonist, publisher and Aviation School trainer, ex- moderator on Medico.in, banker, student councilor ,travelogue writer … among other things! One fine morning, she decided that she had enough of killing herself by Degrees and went back to her first love -- writing. It's more enjoyable! She already has 48 published academic and 14 fiction- in- different- genre books under her belt.

When she is not designing websites or making Graphic design illustrations for clients she is busy browsing in old bookshops for antique books,-she has a mouthwatering collection of priceless First editions and rare books…including R.L. Stevenson, O.Henry, Dornford Yates, Maurice Walsh, C.N.Williamson, Oppenheim, Sapper, Bartimeus, and the crown of her collection- Dickens "The Old Curiosity Shop," and so on… Just call her "Renaissance Woman" - collecting herbal remedies, acting like Universal Helping Hand/Agony Aunt, or escaping to her dear mountains for a bit of exploring, collecting herbs, and plants and trekking.

Check out some of the other JD-Biz Publishing books

Gardening Series on Amazon

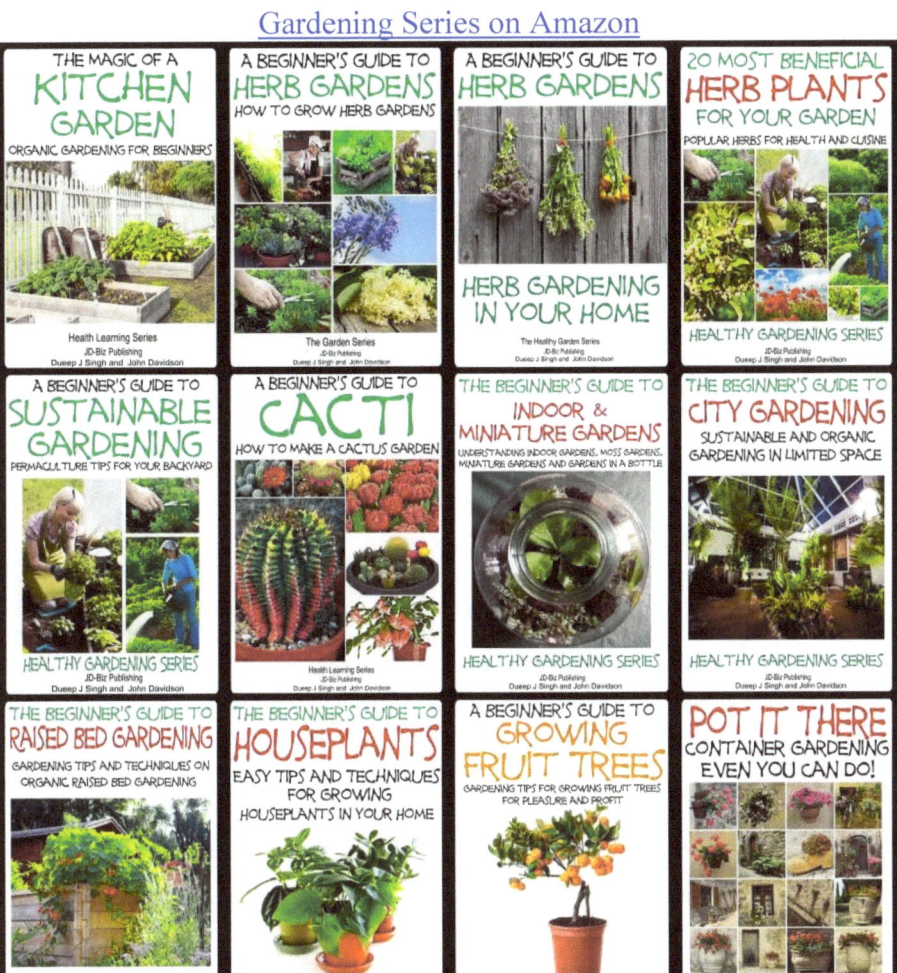

Download Free Books!

http://MendonCottageBooks.com

Health Learning Series

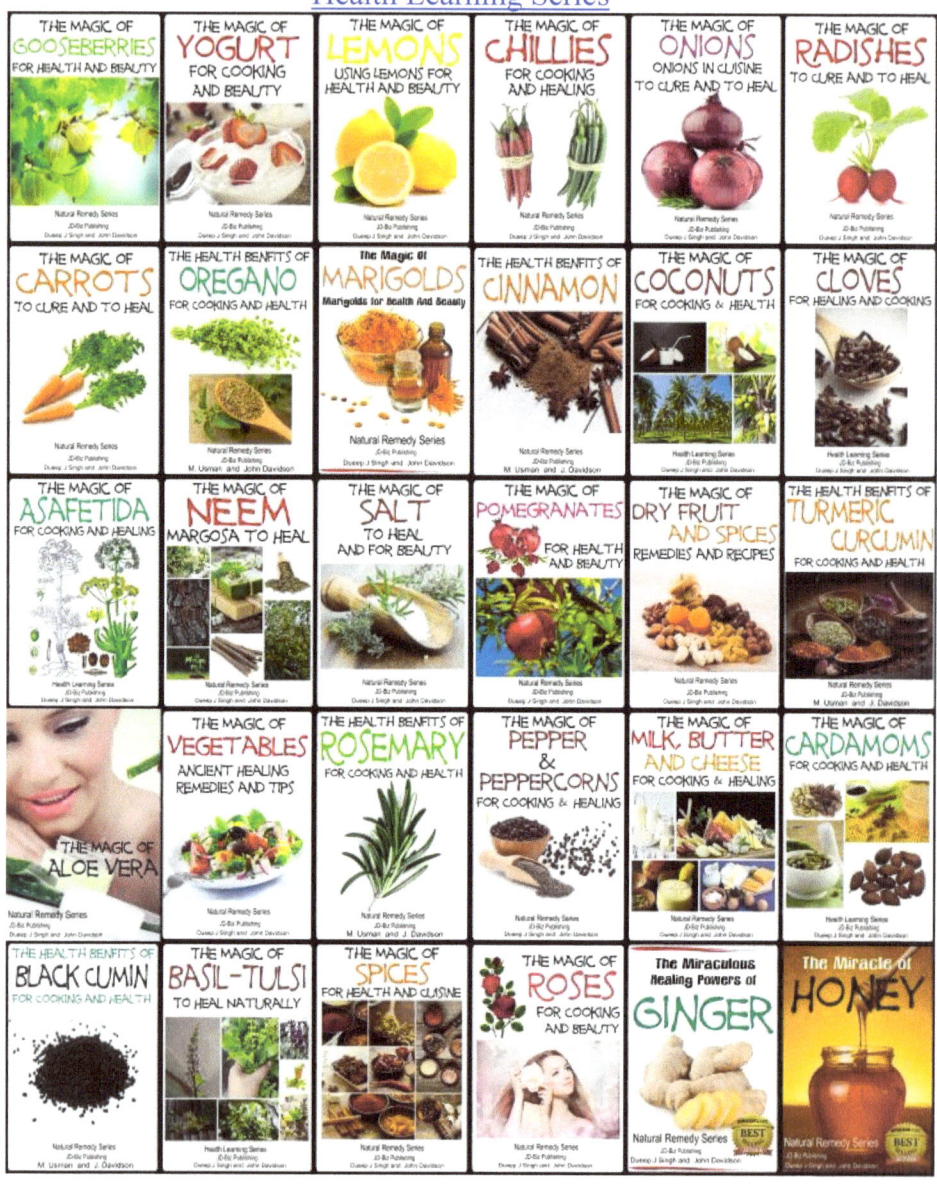

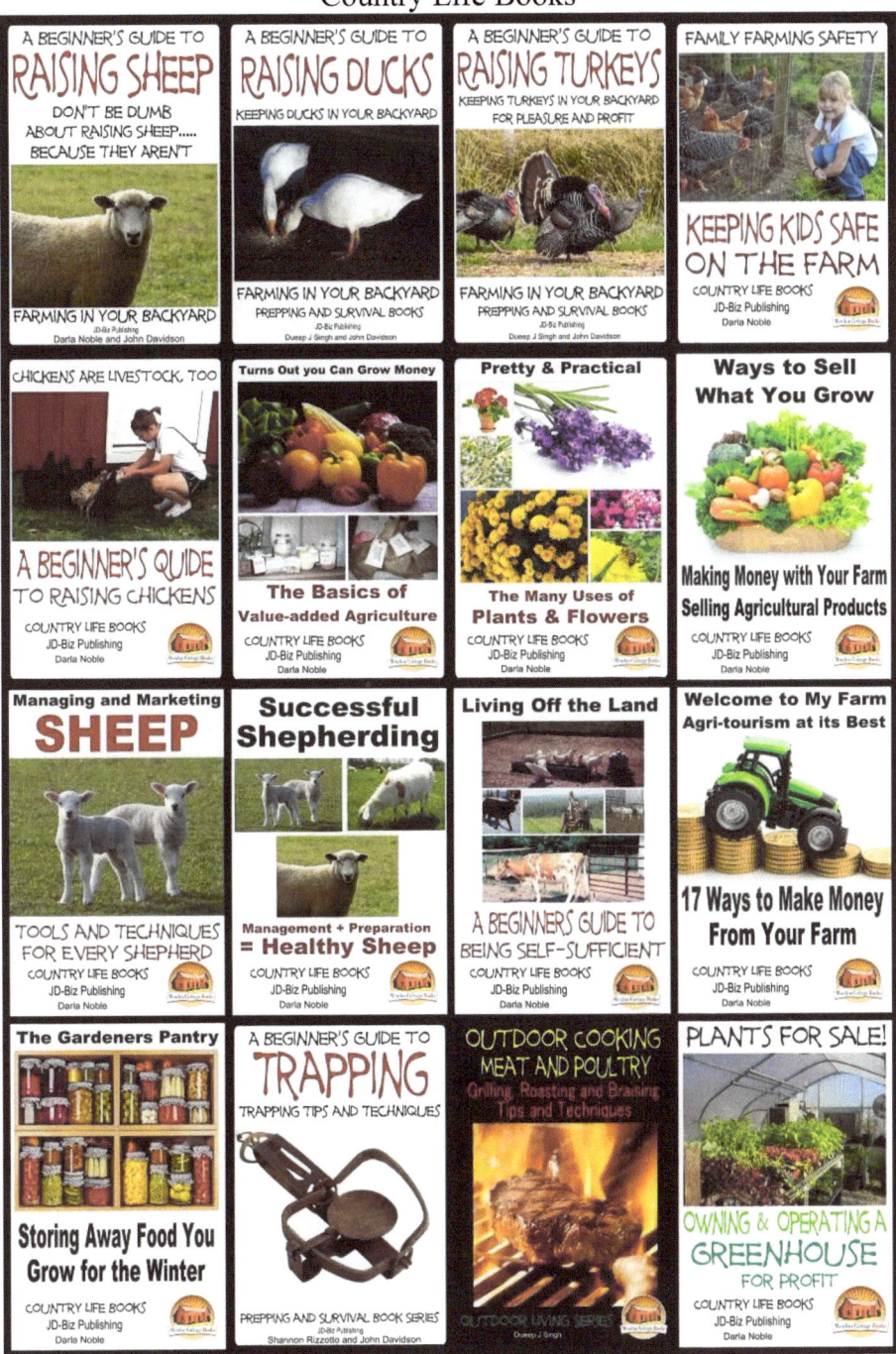

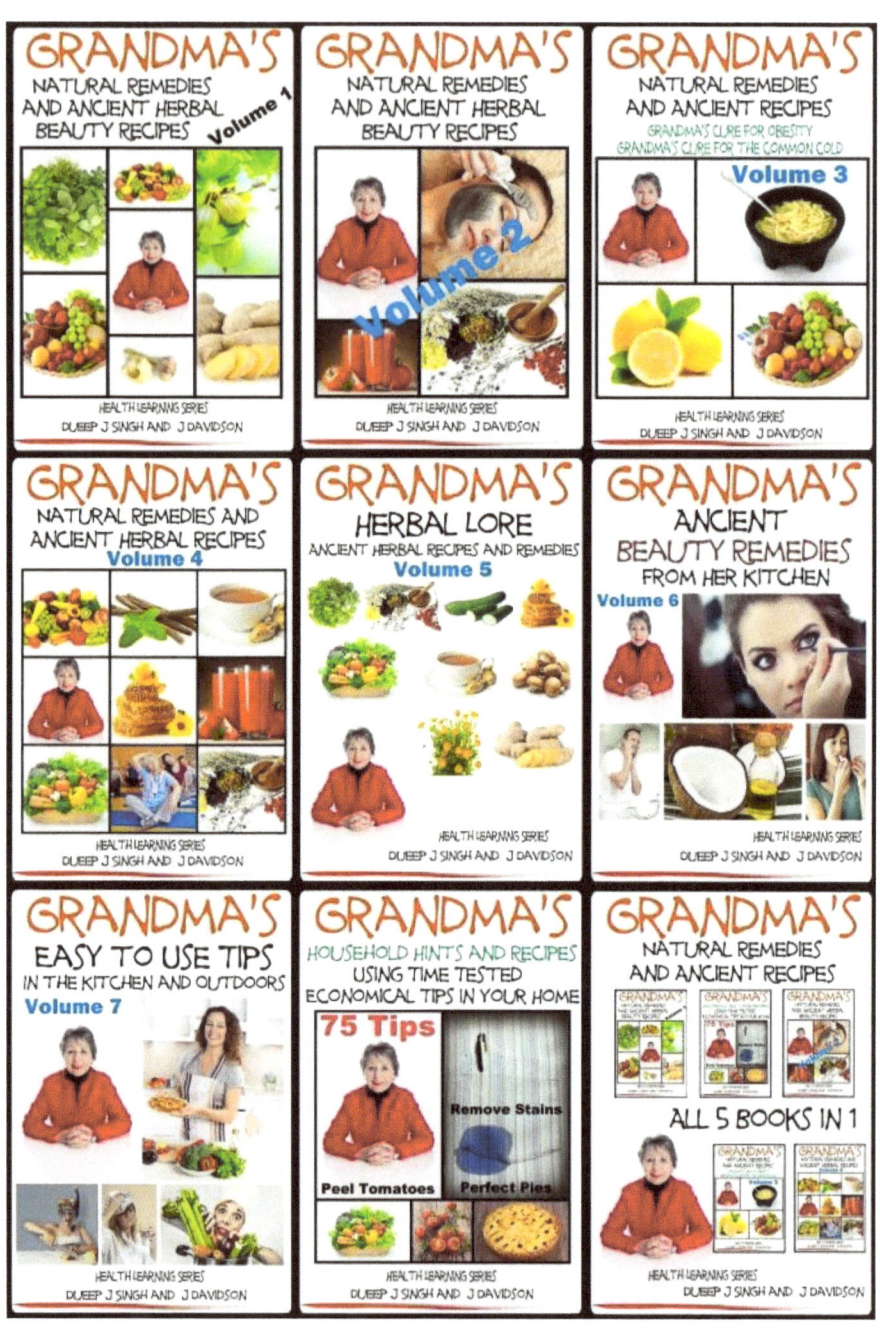

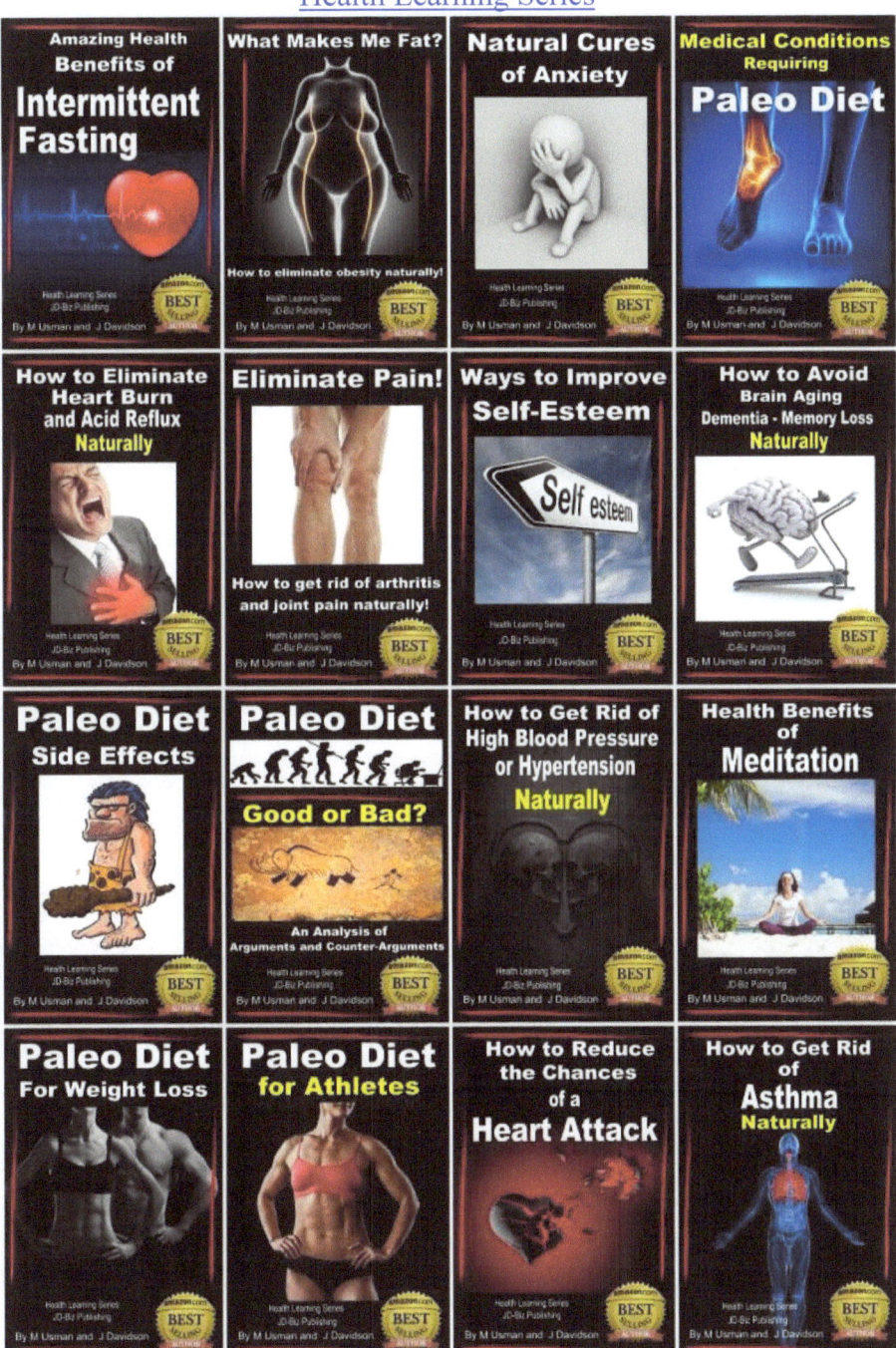

Amazing Animal Book Series

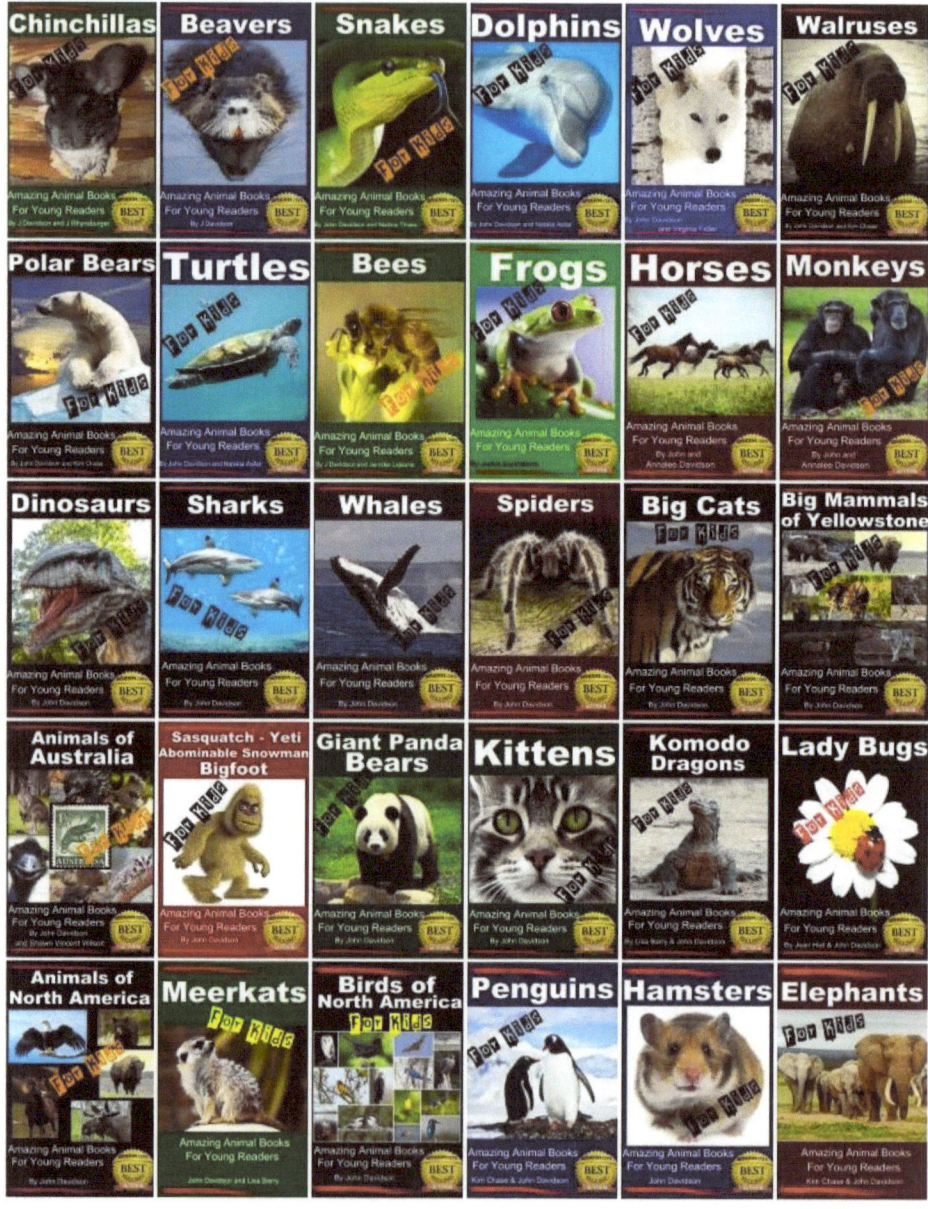

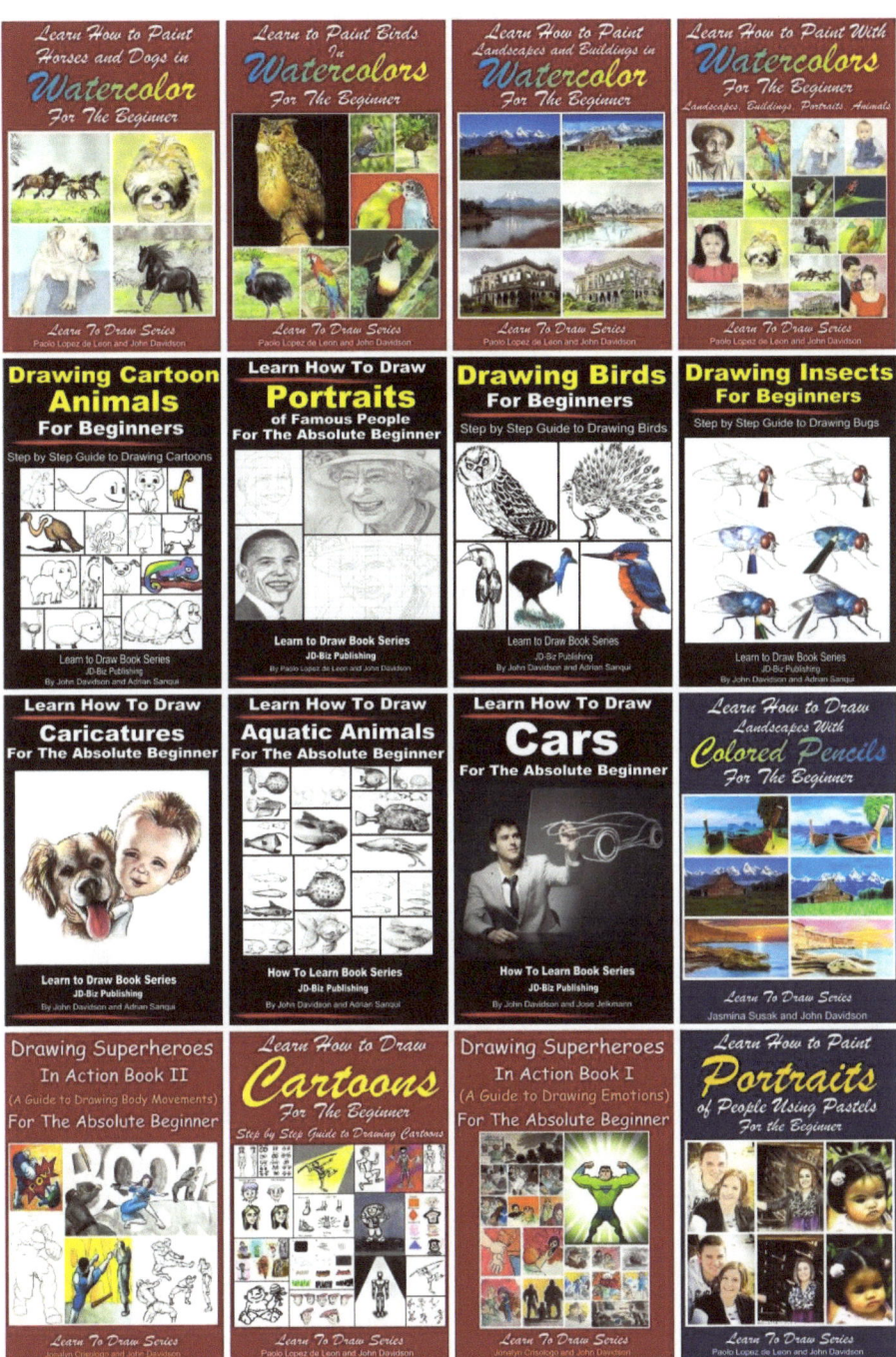

How to Build and Plan Books

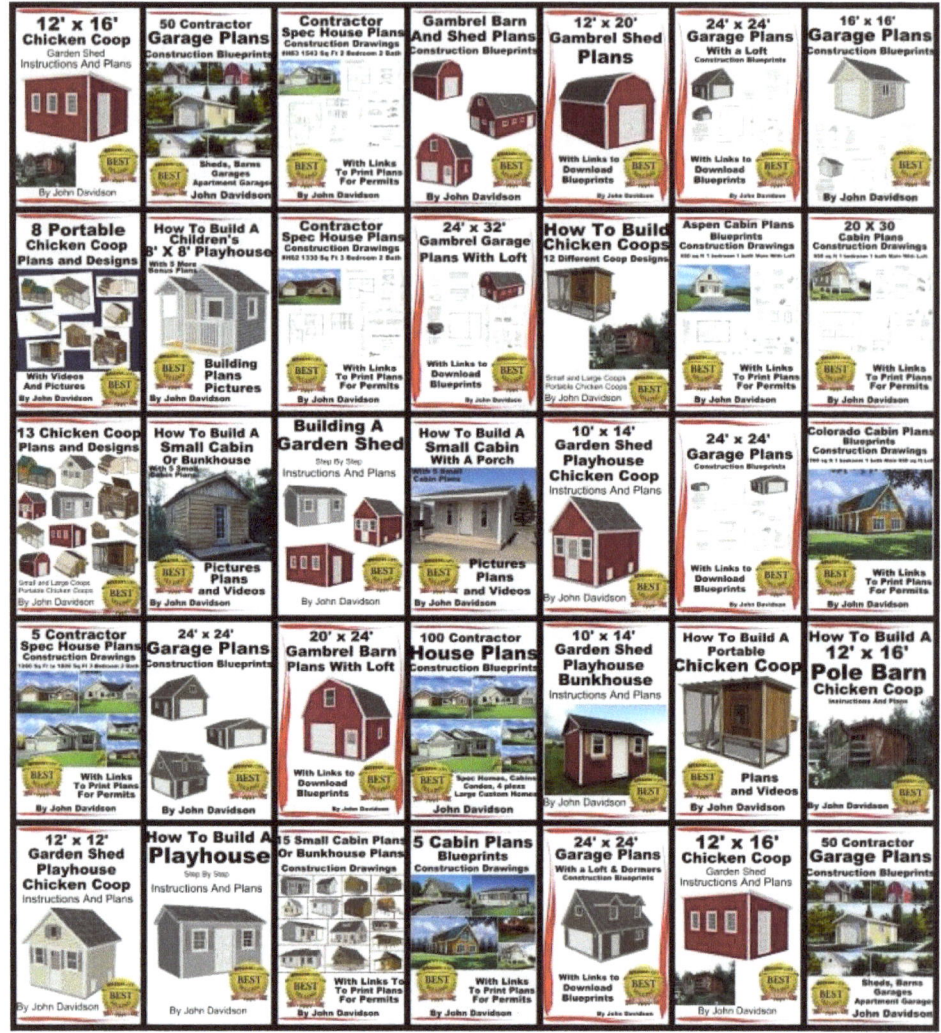

Entrepreneur Book Series

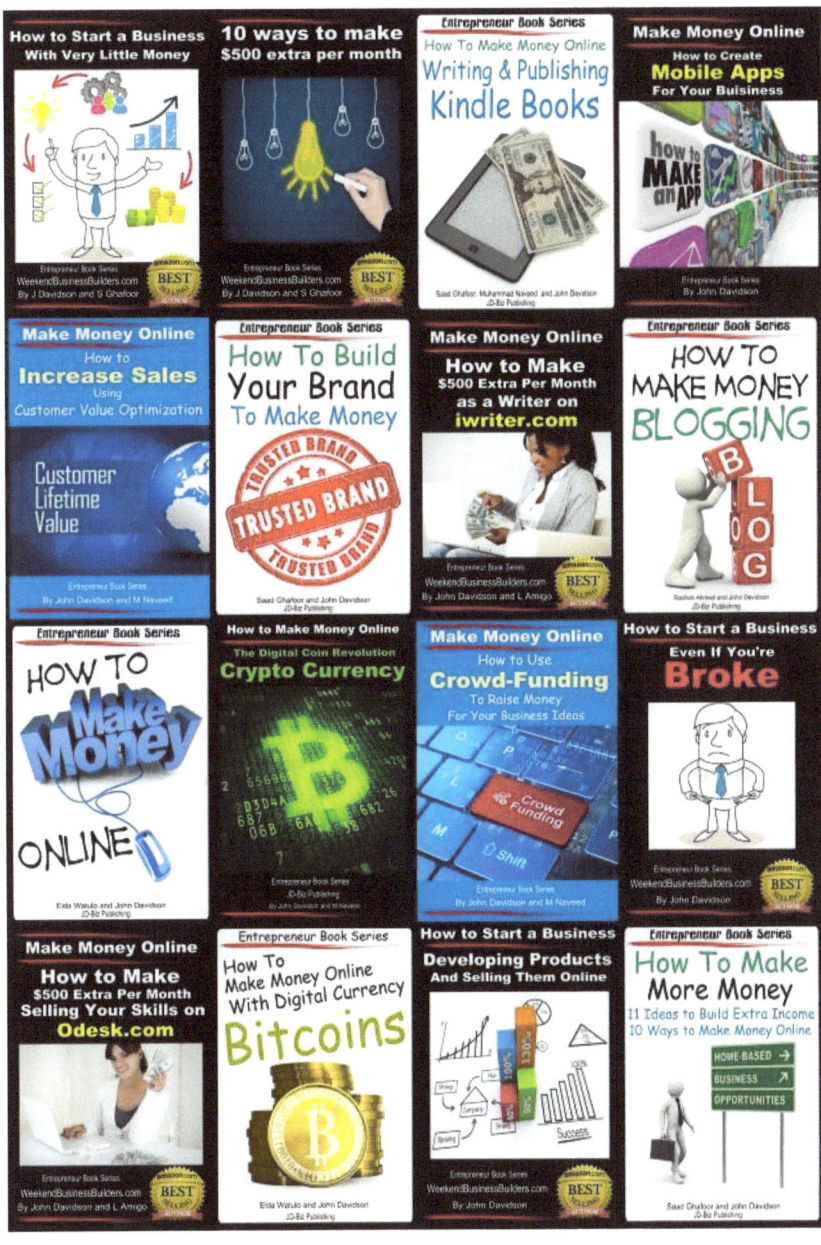

Our books are available at

1. Amazon.com
2. Barnes and Noble
3. Itunes
4. Kobo
5. Smashwords
6. Google Play Books

Download Free Books!

http://MendonCottageBooks.com

Publisher

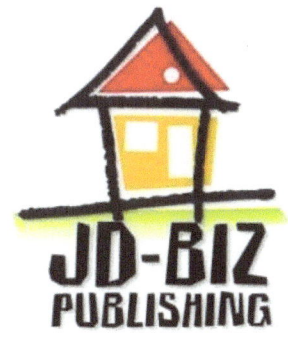

JD-Biz Corp

P O Box 374

Mendon, Utah 84325

http://www.jd-biz.com/

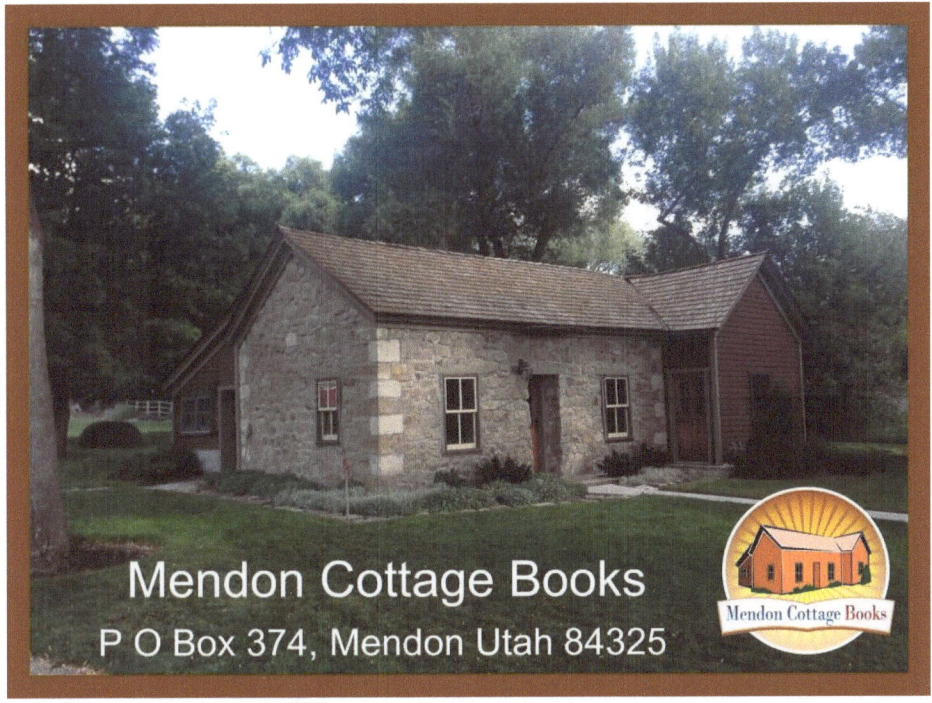

Mendon Cottage Books

P O Box 374, Mendon Utah 84325

www.ingramcontent.com/pod-product-compliance
Lightning Source LLC
Chambersburg PA
CBHW050812290526
45792CB00001B/79